PILATES
ANATOMY

PILATES ANATOMY

Rael Isacowitz

Karen Clippinger

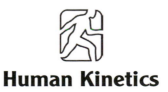

Human Kinetics

Library of Congress Cataloging-in-Publication Data

Isacowitz, Rael, 1955-
  Pilates anatomy / Rael Isacowitz, Karen Clippinger.
    p. cm.
  Includes bibliographical references.
  ISBN-13: 978-0-7360-8386-7 (soft cover)
  ISBN-10: 0-7360-8386-3 (soft cover)
  1. Pilates method. I. Clippinger, Karen S. II. Title.
  RA781.4.I74 2011
  613.7'192--dc22

                              2010046031

ISBN-10: 0-7360-8386-3 (print)
ISBN-13: 978-0-7360-8386-7 (print)

This publication is written and published to provide accurate and authoritative information relevant to the subject matter presented. It is published and sold with the understanding that the author and publisher are not engaged in rendering legal, medical, or other professional services by reason of their authorship or publication of this work. If medical or other expert assistance is required, the services of a competent professional person should be sought.

Acquisitions Editor: Tom Heine; **Developmental Editor:** Cynthia McEntire; **Assistant Editor:** Laura Podeschi; **Copyeditor:** Patricia L. MacDonald; **Graphic Designer:** Fred Starbird; **Graphic Artist:** Francine Hamerski; **Cover Designer:** Keith Blomberg; **Cover Model (for illustration reference):** Lisa Clayton Hubbard; **Photographer (for illustration references):** Neil Bernstein; **Interior Models (for illustration references):** Devon Reuvekamp, Lisa Clayton Hubbard, Stephanie Powel, Yuki Yoshii; **Visual Production Assistant:** Joyce Brumfield; **Art Manager:** Kelly Hendren; **Illustrator:** Molly Borman; **Printer:** Courier Companies, Inc.

Human Kinetics books are available at special discounts for bulk purchase. Special editions or book excerpts can also be created to specification. For details, contact the Special Sales Manager at Human Kinetics.

Printed in the United States of America   10 9 8 7 6 5 4 3 2 1

The paper in this book was manufactured using responsible forestry methods.

Human Kinetics
Web site: www.HumanKinetics.com

United States: Human Kinetics
P.O. Box 5076
Champaign, IL 61825-5076
800-747-4457
e-mail: humank@hkusa.com

Canada: Human Kinetics
475 Devonshire Road Unit 100
Windsor, ON N8Y 2L5
800-465-7301 (in Canada only)
e-mail: info@hkcanada.com

Europe: Human Kinetics
107 Bradford Road
Stanningley
Leeds LS28 6AT, United Kingdom
+44 (0) 113 255 5665
e-mail: hk@hkeurope.com

Australia: Human Kinetics
57A Price Avenue
Lower Mitcham, South Australia 5062
08 8372 0999
e-mail: info@hkaustralia.com

New Zealand: Human Kinetics
P.O. Box 80
Torrens Park, South Australia 5062
0800 222 062
e-mail: info@hknewzealand.com

To Joseph and Clara Pilates and the many dedicated teachers who have kept their vision alive

CONTENTS

PREFACE

In recent years, a profound evolution of Pilates has occurred. The Pilates industry seemed to reach a tipping point (a point of critical mass) in the mid- to late 1990s, whereby it morphed from a little-known form of exercise with a devout but small following including dancers, singers, circus performers, and actors to a mainstream fitness regimen practiced in many households. It suddenly started appearing in Hollywood movies and television commercials, in cartoons and comedy shows, and on late-night television. It became synonymous with going to Starbucks and indulging in a low-fat triple-shot soy latte (no whipped cream please!).

How this happened, why this happened, and to what this phenomenon can be attributed remain somewhat of an enigma. However, few can dispute that the growth of active participants in the United States from approximately 1.7 million in 2000 to approximately 10.6 million in 2006 is a phenomenon. Worldwide participation also has exploded.

Of course, all growth comes with growing pains, and the Pilates industry is no exception. The accelerated education, which is often a part of rapid growth, has certainly taken hold in Pilates. Although we favor a more comprehensive approach, the accelerated approach has been one part of the expansion of Pilates that has led to a multitude of positive outcomes, such as Pilates' filtering into many new arenas including fitness clubs, training programs for athletes, and medical facilities.

Understanding Pilates requires some knowledge of its history. Joseph Pilates was born on December 9, 1883, near Düsseldorf, Germany. He died on October 9, 1967. Unfortunately he didn't live to see the realization of his dreams. He adamantly believed that his approach to total well-being should be embraced by the masses and certainly by health care professionals. He hoped that *contrology,* as he called his system, would be taught in schools throughout the United States. He intended his method to be a mainstream form of conditioning for men, and initially it was practiced more by men, although it is largely women who have kept the flame alive all these years.

It is fortunate that several early students of Mr. Pilates and his wife, Clara, whom he met on his second trip to the United States in 1926 and who became his lifelong partner in his work, survived them and became exceptional teachers in their own right. These first-generation Pilates teachers, taught directly by Joseph and Clara Pilates, have played a profound role in the evolution of the Pilates industry. Rael Isacowitz has had the distinct privilege of studying with several members of this unique group over the past 30 years. Ms. Kathleen Stanford Grant must be singled out as having a particularly powerful effect on this author's development and teaching style.

Joseph Pilates did not leave extensive written materials to guide future generations of Pilates professionals. The limited archival material—photographs, films, and texts—have been very valuable. However, mainly word of mouth and the universal language of movement have been used to pass much of his teachings down from first generation to second and on to following generations. Mr. Pilates did write two short books, and one of them, *Return to Life Through Contrology,* served as the primary reference for *Pilates Anatomy.* The decision to use the exercises as they appear in *Return to Life Through Contrology* as the basis for the primary descriptions of most exercises in *Pilates Anatomy* was an important one. Our goal is for *Pilates Anatomy* to transcend teaching styles, individual approaches to Pilates, or any particular school of Pilates. This book is written to be universal in its appeal, just as anatomy itself is universal. Using *Return to Life Through Contrology* brings the work as close to the source as one can get, with the intent that *Pilates Anatomy* can serve as a bridge for the many different approaches to Pilates that have emerged and can offer a meeting ground for all Pilates professionals and enthusiasts from every part of the Pilates spectrum and all corners of the globe.

Today Pilates can be found in every conceivable environment. Pilates is taught in private studios, academic institutions, fitness centers, and medical facilities. It is used with clients ranging from elite athletes to people with limited capacities due to disease or injury. Age groups ranging from kindergartners to folks in their 90s enjoy the benefits of Pilates. Is there another method that can accommodate such a wide variety of users? This is the magic of Pilates. It is so extremely adaptable. This is certainly one of the reasons for the boom in popularity.

Pilates Anatomy is the work of two authors with much in common but with different expertise to bring to this book. Over the past 30 years, Rael Isacowitz has done extensive study in Pilates, which has included work with the most highly respected early Pilates teachers. He developed an acclaimed Pilates center, and for the last 21 years has designed and directed an internationally renowned Pilates education organization. His knowledge and skill has earned him invitations to travel the world teaching and lecturing. Karen Clippinger has 30 years' experience in teaching anatomy at prominent centers and universities. Her keen ability to make anatomical concepts applicable is well known and has led to her lecturing internationally at many prestigious venues. In the last 17 years, her work has emphasized bringing Pilates to rehabilitation and academic settings, establishing her as a leader in the field. Both of them have rich backgrounds in exercise science and substantial experience as dancers and athletes. Combined they have more than 60 years' experience in study, performance, practice, and teaching, and philosophically they share much in common. Their paths crossed more than 17 years ago, and they have enjoyed a vibrant, often spirited, and always inspiring professional dialogue ever since.

Traveling extensively, presenting, and teaching in many parts of the world gave them a firsthand international perspective on how Pilates is being embraced in so many countries. From China to Russia, from Australia to South Africa, and from the United States to Europe, they have connected with people and contributed to the growth of the industry. There are few countries today in which Pilates is not present. They hope *Pilates Anatomy* will serve as a tool to connect Pilates professionals and enthusiasts alike as an international community speaking an international language.

The direction the expansion of Pilates has taken demands that Pilates professionals have sound knowledge of anatomy. Yet everyone should be able to benefit from the information in this book. The *Pilates Anatomy* approach is designed to be inclusive and not exclusive of any school of Pilates teaching, offering basic anatomical exercise descriptions that can be applied easily to different variations or modifications used by a given approach or for a specific participant. It should be useful for beginning students as well as for physical therapists and others with extensive knowledge of human anatomy. The complementary use of drawings showing targeted working muscles, lists of key muscles, and anatomical information within technique cues and exercise notes will allow the reader to use the information at different levels, in accordance with current knowledge and movement experience. The intention is to offer everyone a solid anatomically based foundation on which to practice Pilates with integrity. Most important, be safe and enjoy!

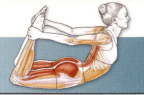
SIX KEY PRINCIPLES OF PILATES

Pilates is not just exercise. Pilates is not just a random choice of particular movements. Pilates is a system of physical and mental conditioning that can enhance your physical strength, flexibility, and coordination as well as reduce stress, improve mental focus, and foster an improved sense of well-being. Pilates can be for anyone and everyone.

Before exploring the anatomy of Pilates, it is important to note that many different approaches to this system have evolved. Some forms of Pilates focus primarily on the physical aspect of the system; others emphasize the mind–body angle. In its original form, Pilates, as expressed emphatically by Joseph H. Pilates, was a system designed to be integrated into every facet of life. Film footage shows Joseph Pilates not only demonstrating exercises and physical activity but also advising on everyday activities such as how to sleep and wash. Although the majority of this book will be devoted to breaking down the muscular involvement in every movement and analyzing each exercise on this basis, it would be an injustice to the system (originally called *contrology*), its founder, and the industry not to address the principles of the method and the mind–body connection.

Foundation Principles of Pilates

Although Joseph Pilates did not specifically notate tenets for his method, the following principles can be identified clearly throughout the pages of his texts and gleaned from original film footage and other archival material. Depending on the school of Pilates, the list of principles and the way they are presented may vary slightly; however, this list—breath, concentration, center, control, precision, and flow—includes those principles that form the basis of many approaches of Pilates and are generally accepted as the foundation of the system.

Breath

Although all the foundation principles share equal importance, the importance of breath and its numerous implications can be observed far beyond the fundamental and crucial role of respiration. This inclusive view is the basis of some approaches to the study of Pilates, but certainly not all. In this context, breath can be described as the fuel of the powerhouse, which is the engine that drives Pilates. It may be viewed as being of the body, of the mind, and of the spirit, as Joseph Pilates regarded it. In this view breath can serve as a common thread that runs through all the foundation principles, in a sense sewing them together.

Breath is one of the keys to life itself—the respiratory muscles are the only *skeletal* muscles essential to life—and yet breath is so often taken for granted. An understanding of the anatomy underlying breath can facilitate optimal use of breath. Because of the complex anatomical processes involved in breathing, breath will be dealt with in greater depth later in this chapter.

Concentration

Concentration can be defined as direction of attention to a single objective, in this case the mastery of a given Pilates exercise. A Pilates practitioner's intent is to perform the exercises as correctly as his or her current skill level will allow. This requires concentration. Begin by going through a mental checklist of points to focus on for each exercise. This may take a few seconds or even a minute or two and should include awareness of the breath pattern as well as the muscles that are about to be worked. Concentrate on the alignment of the body and on maintaining correct alignment and stabilization throughout the execution of the exercise. Maintain mental concentration for the duration of the session.

Center

The concept of center can have several levels of meaning. Primarily it relates to the body's center of gravity. The body's center of gravity is the single point about which every particle of its mass is equally distributed—the point at which the body could be suspended and where it would be totally balanced in all directions.

Each person is built differently and has an individual center of gravity. Where the center of gravity lies distinctly affects how an exercise feels and how difficult or easy it is to execute. Therefore it is a mistake to assume a person lacks strength if he cannot execute an exercise successfully. Lack of success may have more to do with how the person is built and the distribution of body weight. When standing upright with the arms down by the sides, the center of gravity of the average person is located just in front of the second sacral vertebra and at about 55 percent of the person's height. However, significant variances can be observed within, as well as between, genders.

Center also relates to the core and the muscles of the core. In Pilates this is referred to as the *powerhouse,* which will be discussed in greater depth in chapter 2. Center also may have a more esoteric connotation, referring to a feeling of balance within or the eternal spring of energy from which all movement emanates.

Control

Control can be defined as the regulation of the execution of a given action. Refining control is inherent in mastering a skill. The first time someone executes an exercise, he or she has to use control, but as skill increases, this control will be more refined. You can see a distinct difference when viewing a movement performed by someone who has achieved a high level of control and someone who has not. Often a higher level of control is associated with fewer and smaller errors, exact alignment, greater coordination, greater balance, and greater ability to reproduce the exercise successfully over multiple attempts, using less effort and avoiding excessive muscle tension. Refined control requires a great deal of practice, which can aid in developing the necessary strength and flexibility of key muscles as well as allow for the development of more refined motor programs. This practice can also allow these motor programs to run with less conscious attention, so that attention can be paid to finer details and to making minute adjustments, only when needed.

Precision

Precision is key when distinguishing Pilates from many other exercise systems. Precision can be described as the exact manner in which an action is executed. Often the exercise itself is not so different from other exercise regimens, but the way it is executed is different.

Knowledge of anatomy aids greatly in achieving precision. You will understand which muscles are working or should be working. You will align your body correctly and understand the goals of an exercise. The greater the precision, the more likely the goal will be achieved and the greater the benefit from doing the exercise. Precision is key to the Pilates approach to movement and to the infinite corrections that need to be implemented through the learning process.

Precision can be associated with the activation of isolated muscles and at the same time with the integration of the required muscles to create movement. Precision can make the difference between accessing a muscle or not and between achieving the goal or not.

Flow

Flow is an essential quality to strive for. Flow can be described as a smooth, uninterrupted continuity of movement. Romana Kryzanowska describes the Pilates method as "flowing motion outward from a strong center." Flow requires a deep understanding of the movement and incorporates precise muscle activation and timing. As movement proficiency develops from extensive practice, each movement and each session should flow.

Some approaches also encourage a more esoteric use of flow. This meaning is exemplified in the statement by Mihály Csíkszentmihályi that "flow is the mental state of operation in which the person is fully immersed in what he or she is doing by a feeling of energized focus, full involvement, and success in the process of the activity."

These six elements should be present when executing the exercises in this book and throughout daily activities. The common denominator of the six principles is that each one has a distinct physical and mental component. These very elements connect the body and the mind and permit the anatomical understanding to which this book is largely devoted to have a greater impact on your life.

The way in which each person integrates these principles into the practice of Pilates and life itself is individual. For example, one person may emphasize more of the physical aspects, using Pilates to enhance athletic performance, improve muscle tone, or aid with recovery from injury. Another person may place greater import on the mental aspects, using Pilates to reduce stress or aid with improving focus and concentration in his or her life. Yet the important issue is that the execution of each exercise and the practice of the system as a whole are not just a careless imitation of the illustrated exercise steps provided in this book, but rather a process focused on learning how the exercises are executed and applying these six principles in accordance with your current physical and mental acuity.

A Closer Look at the Science of Breathing

Breath is the first principle mentioned in this chapter and one that, historically, has played a vital role in most mind–body systems. It is accepted by many Pilates professionals as having paramount importance in the practice of the method. Discussions and, at times, disagreements as to a particular breath pattern, or whether a set breath pattern is necessary at all, may arise. However, few people would dispute the importance of breath for exercise, and a better understanding of breathing can help you obtain greater benefits from the exercises in this book.

The major function of the respiratory system is to deliver oxygen to and remove carbon dioxide from the tissues of the body. Although every cell in the body must have oxygen to live, the body's need to rid itself of carbon dioxide, a by-product of cellular metabolism, is the most important stimulus for breathing in a healthy person. At least four processes are involved, collectively termed *respiration.* The first two processes, *external respiration,* involve movement of external air into the lungs (pulmonary ventilation) and from the lungs into the blood (pulmonary diffusion), and vice versa. This book will focus on these first two processes. The next two processes involve the transport of gases by the circulatory system to tissues such as muscles and the exchange of oxygen and carbon dioxide between the capillary blood and tissue cells.

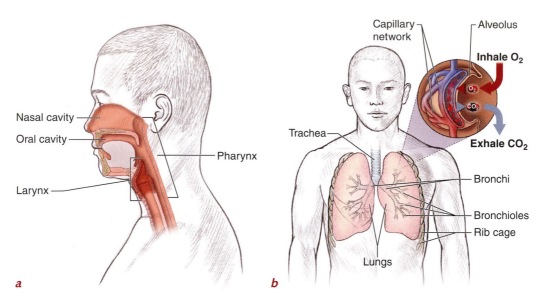

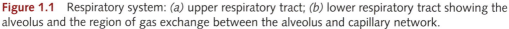

Figure 1.1   Respiratory system: *(a)* upper respiratory tract; *(b)* lower respiratory tract showing the alveolus and the region of gas exchange between the alveolus and capillary network.

Anatomy of the Respiratory System

The lungs of an average-size person weigh about 2.2 pounds (1 kg). They are compact and fit within the thoracic cavity. However, because of the extensive network of tubes and millions of gas-filled air spaces (alveoli), if spread out the tissue would occupy a surface area about the size of a singles tennis court or a medium-size swimming pool. This unique structure provides the lungs with a massive surface area that is ideal for their vital function of gas exchange.

Structurally, the respiratory system can be divided into two major parts—the upper and lower respiratory tracts. The upper respiratory tract (figure 1.1a) is a system of interconnecting cavities and tubes (nasal cavity, oral cavity, pharynx, and larynx) that provide a pathway for the air into the lower respiratory tract. This upper tract also serves to purify, warm, and humidify the air before it reaches the final portion of the lower tract. The lower respiratory tract (trachea, bronchi, bronchioles, and alveoli, figure 1.1b) terminates in structures that allow for the exchange of gases, including approximately 300 million alveoli and their associated extensive network of capillaries. The wall of an alveolus is thinner than a piece of tissue paper, easily allowing for oxygen to pass from the alveolus into the tiny pulmonary capillaries and for carbon dioxide to pass from the pulmonary capillaries into the alveolus by simple diffusion.

Mechanics of Breathing

Pulmonary ventilation, commonly termed *breathing,* consists of two phases. The process of moving air into the lungs is called *inhalation* or *inspiration,* and the process of moving gases out of the lungs is called *exhalation* or *expiration.* In essence, pulmonary ventilation is a mechanical process that involves volume changes in the thoracic cavity that lead to pressure changes, which result in the flow of gases to equalize pressures. The changes in volume necessary for pressure changes are greatly aided by the structure of the thorax (sternum, ribs with associated cartilages, and vertebrae). The ribs articulate with the spine so that they can move upward and outward during inspiration and downward and inward during expiration.

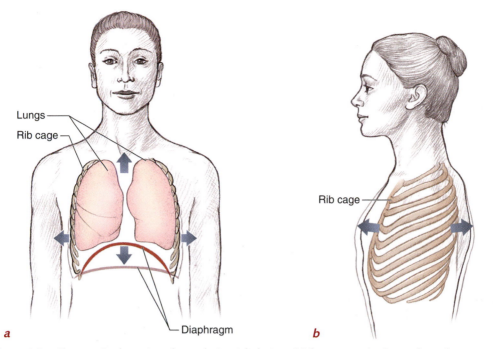

Figure 1.2   Changes in thoracic volume during inhalation: *(a)* front view displaying lateral expansion in the lower thorax due to orientation of ribs and contraction of the diaphragm; *(b)* side view displaying forward and backward expansion in the upper thorax due to orientation of ribs and sternum.

Inhalation

Inhalation (inspiration) is initiated by activation of the respiratory muscles, particularly the diaphragm. When the dome-shaped diaphragm contracts, it flattens out, allowing more height in the thoracic cavity (figure 1.2*a*). The external intercostals act to lift the rib cage and pull the sternum forward. The orientation of the ribs is such that the ribs of the midthorax and lower thorax increase volume more laterally, or sideways, while the ribs of the upper thoracic cavity increase thoracic volume more in a forward and backward direction (figure 1.2*b*). The increase in volume of the thoracic cavity produced by these respiratory muscles results in the pressure within the alveoli of the lungs (intrapulmonary pressure) being lower than the outside atmospheric pressure. Thus, air enters the lungs until the intrapulmonary pressure is equal to the atmospheric pressure (the pressure exerted by the air outside the body).

The expansion of the lungs is also aided by an additional mechanism relating to the surface tension between two important membranes. These two thin membranes are called *pleurae*. The *visceral pleura* covers the lungs, and the *parietal pleura* covers the inside of the chest wall and diaphragm. Between these two pleurae, the pleural space exists. It is airtight and contains a small amount of fluid. As the chest wall expands, the lungs are drawn outward, coupling the outer covering of the lungs with the inner lining of the thorax wall because of the increase of the negative pressure in the pleural space.

When pulmonary ventilation demands increase, such as during rigorous exercise or with some pulmonary diseases, the two previously described processes are aided by activation of many other accessory muscles. During inspiration, for example, additional muscles such as the scalenes, sternocleidomastoid, pectoralis major, and pectoralis minor can be recruited to help further elevate the ribs. Muscles such as the erector spinae can help straighten the thoracic curve so that a greater increase in thoracic volume precipitates a greater volume of incoming air.

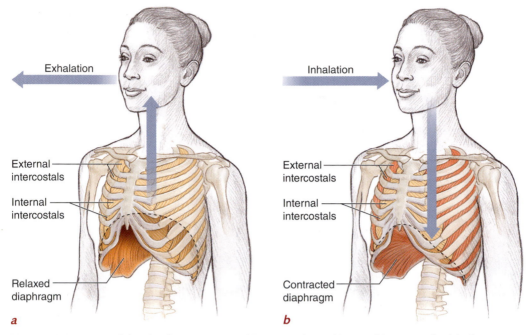

Exhalation

External intercostals

Internal intercostals

Relaxed diaphragm

a

Inhalation

External intercostals

Internal intercostals

Contracted diaphragm

b

Figure 1.3   Action of the diaphragm, external intercostals, and internal intercostals: *(a)* after passive exhalation, showing the diaphragm in a dome shape and the external intercostals and internal intercostals relaxed; *(b)* during inhalation, displaying the diaphragm contracted (flattened), external intercostals contracted, and internal intercostals relaxed.

Exhalation

Exhalation (expiration) with quiet breathing is primarily passive, relying on the elastic recoil of the lung tissue and changes associated with relaxation of the respiratory muscles. As the diaphragm relaxes, it moves upward into the thorax. The ribs lower as the intercostal muscles relax (figure 1.3). The thoracic cavity volume decreases. This, in turn, increases the intrapulmonary pressure relative to the outside atmospheric pressure, resulting in air flowing from the lungs to outside the body.

However, when exhalation is forced, such as when pulmonary ventilation requirements increase, active contraction of many muscles can be added to the passive mechanisms. For example, contraction of the abdominal muscles can press the diaphragm upward via intra-abdominal pressure as well as aid other muscles such as the internal intercostals, quadratus lumborum, and latissimus dorsi in depressing the rib cage.

Breathing During the Practice of Pilates

The belief that breathing exercises, or voluntarily controlled breathing patterns, may provide health benefits or enhance physical performance has been shared by many cultures for centuries. The proposed benefits range from enhanced relaxation and decreased stress to lowered blood pressure, improved focus, activation of specific muscles, better circulation and respiration, and even lowered risk for cardiovascular disease. Although some scientific research exists regarding the potential positive effects of various controlled breathing techniques, additional research is needed to better understand these benefits and create optimal training techniques. However, one cannot ignore the number of disciplines, both Eastern and Western, that use breath in a profound way—yoga, tai chi, aikido, karate, capoeira, dance, swimming, weightlifting, and so on. Some systems of training have endeavored to harness different effects of breath to enhance performance or foster health of the body, mind, and spirit.

Pilates uses breathing in various ways in an attempt to foster these greater benefits. Three key ways that breathing is shaped, or controlled, in Pilates is through lateral breathing, set breath patterns, and active breathing.

Lateral Breathing

Lateral, or *intercostal, breathing* emphasizes the lateral expansion of the rib cage while maintaining a consistent inward pull of the deep abdominal muscles during both inhalation and exhalation (figure 1.4). This is in contrast to the type of breathing that emphasizes the lowering of the diaphragm during inhalation (often called *diaphragmatic breathing*), with the abdominal muscles relaxed so they are allowed to push outward.

A reason for using lateral breathing is to help maintain abdominal contraction while performing Pilates exercises during which keeping a stable core is important for successful performance and for protection of the body. This by no means implies that diaphragmatic breathing is negative or that the diaphragm does not still play a vital role in breathing, only that lateral breathing is the preferred mode during the practice of Pilates.

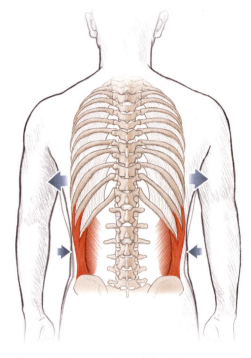

Figure 1.4 Expansion of the rib cage during inhalation when using lateral breathing, with a corsetlike action around the middle trunk for support.

Set Breath Patterns

The Pilates exercises in this book have a set breath pattern. An inhalation occurs during some phase of the movement, and an exhalation occurs during another phase. One reason for these patterns is to keep you from holding your breath, particularly when a lot of effort is required in an exercise. Holding the breath can be associated with excessive muscle tension and an undesired and potentially dangerous increase in blood pressure (the Valsalva maneuver). Exhaling during the phase that requires greater exertion can prevent holding the breath.

A given breath pattern may also influence the muscles being recruited. For example, an exhalation can foster activation of the deep abdominal muscle called the transversus abdominis, discussed in chapter 2.

Lastly, the breath pattern can help establish the dynamic, or rhythm, of a given Pilates exercise. Every exercise in Pilates has a particular quality. Some exercises or phases of a given exercise are performed more slowly and smoothly. Others are performed more rapidly and forcefully. The varying dynamics assist in giving a Pilates session variety as well as simulating daily activities more closely.

Active Breathing

A special case in which breathing may dramatically influence the dynamic of an exercise is active breathing. In signature exercises such as Hundred, the breath is pushed out not only more forcefully during exhalation but also with a percussive emphasis as the practitioner actively contracts the abdominals and particularly the internal intercostals in stages. On the inhale, the breath is drawn in with a percussive emphasis in stages, highlighting the external intercostals. Hundred, for example, requires five beats during inhalation and five beats during exhalation. Each beat represents further contraction of these muscles.

Use of active breathing should be individual. People who work with excessive tension are encouraged to use a more relaxed and softer mode of breathing. For some, active breathing may help activate target muscles and inject a higher energy into a Pilates session.

Ron Fletcher, an early student of Joseph and Clara Pilates and one of the foremost teachers of Pilates, developed an approach to breathing called Percussive Breathing. He explains: "The breath shapes the movement and defines its dynamic." *Percussive* should not be mistaken for *forceful;* rather, it offers a sound and rhythm to the breath that fluctuates with each exercise. Think of it as inflating a balloon and then releasing as much air as possible through a small opening in a constant, steady stream. This concept is reminiscent of Joseph Pilates' breathometer, a spinning wheel that turned as one blew at it. The goal was to keep the wheel turning at a consistent velocity. "There needs to be intention to both the inhale and exhale," Fletcher notes, recalling Joseph Pilates saying in his thick German accent, "You must out the air before you can in the air." Fletcher adds, "Inspiration is inspiration for the movement."

Application of Foundation Principles to Mat Work

Mat work forms the foundation of Pilates, not only in terms of the exercises but also in terms of the practice and integration of the principles into the work and into your life. The foundation principles should be present throughout your practice of Pilates in order to produce maximum results. Follow these steps while learning and mastering the exercises.

First focus on learning the basic movement pattern based on the breath pattern described in each exercise. Closely note the positions of the body shown in the illustrations, and read the descriptions.

Use keen concentration when practicing the movement to help achieve the sense of center and control associated with making a movement second nature through the development of an easily recalled, accurate, and reliable motor program. Focus on the cues (and feel free to add more of your own) to aid in achieving the precision inherent in Pilates. Practice the movement pattern until you become familiar with the many nuances of the movement. Each movement demands intricate timing and activation of the correct muscles in a particular recruitment pattern.

As you master the timing and apply all the principles, the quality of flow will be born in the movement. At this point you may pay attention to the transitions from one movement to the next. This helps create a general flow in your workout as a whole.

Combining the foundation principles of Pilates with a deeper understanding of the workings of the body though the anatomical information in the upcoming pages is a powerful combination and one that will certainly bring with it a multitude of benefits. A key to success lies in practice. With consistent practice and reinforcement of the movements, you will undoubtedly enjoy the wonderful world of Pilates.

SPINE, CORE, AND BODY ALIGNMENT

Body alignment can be described as the relative positioning of body segments, such as placement of the head relative to the shoulders. *Static alignment* is this relative positioning when the body is stationary. The relative positioning that occurs during movement is *dynamic alignment.* Both static and dynamic alignment are important in Pilates. Pilates should improve awareness of body alignment as well as your ability to achieve the desired body alignment associated with a given movement or position.

The Skeleton

To understand and improve alignment, we need to look deep inside the body at the structural building blocks—the 206 bones of the human skeleton—that help determine alignment. The skeleton has two major divisions: the axial skeleton and the appendicular skeleton. As seen in figure 2.1 on page 10, the *axial skeleton* (in yellow) is made up of the skull, vertebral column (spine), ribs, and sternum (breastbone). As its name suggests, when standing, the axial skeleton forms the central upright axis of the body to which the limbs are attached.

The *appendicular* skeleton consists of the bones that make up the limbs, or appendages. The appendicular skeleton has two subdivisions: the paired upper extremities and the paired lower extremities. Each of the two *upper extremities* (shown in green in figure 2.1) contains one clavicle (collarbone); one scapula (shoulder blade); one humerus (upper arm bone); one radius and one ulna (the forearm bones); and eight carpals, five metacarpals, and 14 phalanges (the bones of the hand). Each of the two *lower extremities* (shown in blue in figure 2.1) contains one os coxae (hip bone); one femur (thigh bone); one tibia (shinbone) and one fibula (the smaller bone in the lower leg); and seven tarsals, five metatarsals, and 14 phalanges (the bones of the foot). In the adult, one hip bone, technically termed the *os coxae* or *coxal bone,* is made up of three fused bones: the ilium, ischium, and pubis.

The Essential Spine

The spine provides the primary movements of the axial skeleton. And the movement, stability, and alignment of the spine are an essential focus in Pilates.

Elemental Vertebrae

The spine, or vertebral column, is made up of 33 bones called *vertebrae* that are stacked one upon the next to form a long columnlike structure. As shown in figure 2.2 on page 11, the vertebrae get larger in size from top to bottom as they progress from the neck to the pelvis. The vertebrae are arranged in five regions. The first three regions are depicted in color in figure 2.2 for emphasis, as these three regions contain the 24 vertebrae that are responsible for the primary movements of the spine.

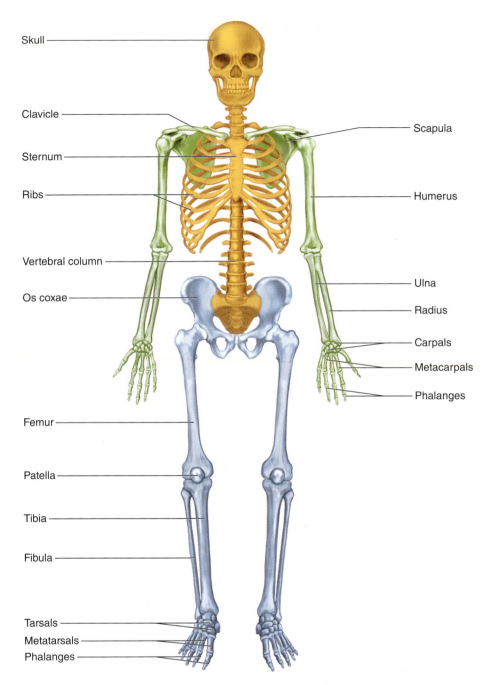

Figure 2.1 Bones of the skeleton (front view). The axial skeleton is in yellow. The two subdivisions of the appendicular skeleton are shown; the upper extremities are in green, and the lower extremities are in blue.

- **Cervical (green).** The top seven vertebrae that span from below the head to the base of the neck are the *cervical vertebrae*. The smallest and lightest vertebrae, they are essential for movements of the head and neck.

- **Thoracic (blue).** The next 12 vertebrae are the *thoracic vertebrae*. They span from just below the neck to the last rib and gradually increase in size from top to bottom. They are unique in that they articulate with the ribs. The thoracic vertebrae are key for movements of the thorax, including the upper back.

- **Lumbar (yellow).** The next five vertebrae are the *lumbar vertebrae*. They span from just below the last rib to the pelvic girdle. These vertebrae are stronger and more massive than those above and are essential for their weight-bearing function. The lumbar vertebrae are important for movements of the lower back.

- **Sacrum.** The next five vertebrae are called the *sacral vertebrae*. Rather than act independently, they are fused in adults to form the triangular-shaped *sacrum*. Each side of the sacrum joins with one hip bone, providing important stability for the pelvis. Because these vertebrae are fused, the primary movements of the sacrum occur relative to the last lumbar vertebrae. This joint between the last lumbar vertebra and the sacrum is called the *lumbosacral joint*. Movements at this joint have a profound influence on alignment of the lower back and pelvis.

- **Coccyx.** The last four (or sometimes three or five) vertebrae are called the *coccygeal vertebrae*. They are fused to form a small triangle that is considered the vestigial tailbone. Hence, these vertebrae are often collectively referred to as the tailbone, although their technical name is the *coccyx*.

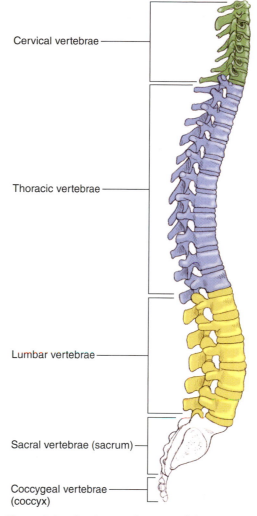

Cervical vertebrae

Thoracic vertebrae

Lumbar vertebrae

Sacral vertebrae (sacrum)

Coccygeal vertebrae (coccyx)

Figure 2.2   Regions and curves of the spine (view of right side of vertebral column).

As can be seen in figure 2.2, the spine is not a straight rod. Instead, each of these regions has a distinct curve when viewed from the side. The cervical and lumbar regions are curved such that they are concave to the back, while the remaining regions are curved such that they are concave to the front. Ideally, these curvatures are each of a normal magnitude and are balanced relative to one another. These curves play an important role in both enhancing movements of the spine and shock absorption.

Joints Between Vertebrae

The lumbar, thoracic, and all but the top two cervical vertebrae are joined to the vertebrae above and below by a series of joints that greatly influence the ranges of motion that are possible between consecutive vertebrae. As shown in figure 2.3, the front rounded portion of each vertebra (the vertebral body) is joined to adjacent vertebrae by an *inter-vertebral disc,* forming a cartilaginous joint. This intervertebral disc has a strong outer ring of fibrous tissue called the *annulus fibro-sus* (shown in gray) and an inner gelatinous central mass, the *nucleus pulposus* (shown in purple). The nucleus pulposus has a high water content, and the discs can be likened to little water cushions between the vertebrae that are vital for shock absorption and protection of the spine.

The back portions of these vertebrae are also connected by little paired joints called *facet joints* that allow small gliding move-ments. The shape and facing of the projec-tions of the vertebrae (the articular processes) that come together to form these facet joints influence the movement allowed in this region of the spine. For example, the facing of the facet joints enhances rotation in the thoracic region but limits rotation in the lumbar region.

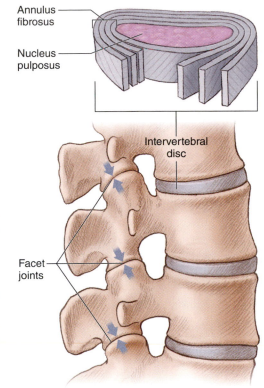

Figure 2.3 Joints of the spine. Facet joints and intervertebral discs, with a detail of an intervertebral disc.

The motion of the vertebral column is also influenced by the presence of many strong bands of fibrous tissue that span between the vertebrae. These ligaments help control how far a vertebra can move in a given direction, provide important stability for the spine, and help prevent forward or backward bulging of the intervertebral discs.

Many factors such as strength imbalances, flexibility imbalances, postural habits, and injuries result in most people having areas in the spine in which movement is restricted, movement is excessive, or movement is asymmetrical. One of the goals of Pilates is to help fully utilize the potential range in each segment of the spine in a symmetrical manner.

Movements of the Spine

The large movements of the spine utilized in Pilates are illustrated in figure 2.4. Spinal *flexion* refers to a forward bending of the spine such as what occurs when rolling the spine down to touch the toes or when curling the upper trunk forward and up into a sit-up; *extension* describes a straightening of the spine from a flexed position or movement backward beyond straight (figure 2.4*a*). The backward movement beyond straight can also be termed spinal *hyperextension.* Bending the spine sideways to the right is called *right lateral flexion,* while bending it back up toward a straight position or to the opposite side is termed *left lateral flexion* (figure 2.4*b*). Rotating the head or upper trunk so that the face or chest faces to the right is called *right rotation,* while rotating the head or upper trunk back to center or toward the other side is termed *left rotation* (figure 2.4*c*).

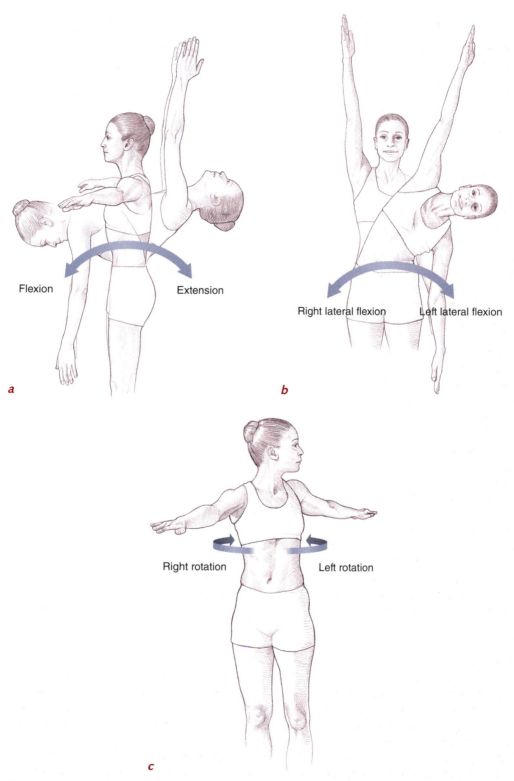

Figure 2.4 Movements of the spine: *(a)* flexion and extension; *(b)* right lateral flexion and left lateral flexion; *(c)* right rotation and left rotation.

Primary Muscles of the Spine

Many muscles of the spine produce movement or affect stability. Two of the most vital muscle groups are the abdominals and spinal extensors. The iliopsoas and quadratus lumborum also are key in certain circumstances.

Abdominals

The abdominals have long been appreciated for their potential to help create a flatter abdomen, enhance movement technique, improve certain postural problems, and reduce the risk for certain types of back injuries. There are four paired abdominal muscles: rectus abdominis, external oblique, internal oblique, and transversus abdominis. All of the abdominals attach into a tendinous band that runs vertically down the center of the abdomen (linea alba), but the location and direction of their muscle fibers are quite different. As seen in figure 2.5a, the rectus abdominis runs straight up and down in the central portion of the abdomen. In contrast, the external oblique runs diagonally downward toward the center, with its muscle fibers located to the side of the rectus abdominis. The internal oblique is deep to the external oblique, and its upper fibers run upward toward the center, with its muscle fibers also lateral to the rectus abdominis.

When both sides of these three abdominals contract simultaneously, they are all capable of producing spinal flexion, with the rectus abdominis being particularly powerful. When one side of these three abdominals contracts, they are all capable of producing lateral flexion to the same side, with the obliques being particularly effective. Contraction of one side of the obliques can also produce rotation, with the external oblique producing rotation to the opposite side and the internal oblique producing rotation to the same side. When you perform a curl-up type of exercise such as Chest Lift (page 54), both sides of all three of these abdominals work to produce the desired flexion of the spine. However, when rotating to the left, as in Chest Lift With Rotation (page 64), only the left external and right internal obliques can produce the desired rotation, while both the right and left rectus abdominis muscles primarily act to maintain the spine lifted off the mat in flexion.

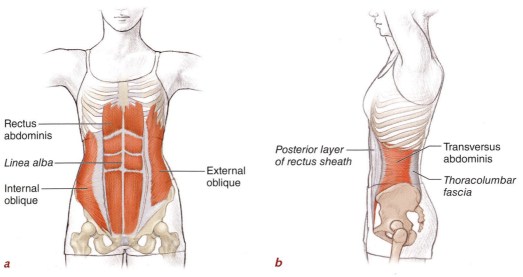

Rectus abdominis

Linea alba

Internal oblique

External oblique

Posterior layer of rectus sheath

Transversus abdominis

Thoracolumbar fascia

a   b

Figure 2.5   Abdominals: *(a)* front view of external oblique and rectus abdominis on left side of body and rectus abdominis and internal oblique on right; *(b)* side view of trunk showing transversus abdominis.

The fourth abdominal muscle, the transversus abdominis (transverse abdominal muscle) is generally the deepest abdominal muscle. Its fibers run in an approximately horizontal direction across the abdomen as seen in figure 2.5b. Hence, it is not capable of producing spinal flexion, although it may assist with rotation. Its primary function is considered postural, and its contraction results in pulling the abdominal wall inward and compressing the abdominal contents similar to a corset. The transversus abdominis has been shown to play an important role in protecting the spine, automatically contracting to help stabilize the healthy spine and pelvis just before movements of the limbs. It can also aid with respiration and is recruited with forced expiration. In Pilates, therefore, an exhalation is sometimes used to encourage its activation. There is a strong emphasis on the use of the transversus abdominis in many current approaches to teaching Pilates.

Spinal Extensors

The paired spinal extensors are located on the back of the trunk, and they share the common action of extending the spine, or back. These vital muscles that at one time were neglected in favor of emphasizing abdominal strength have been shown to be key for optimal movement performance; prevention of certain back injuries, osteoporosis, and certain postural problems; and successful return to activity after back injury. The spinal extensors can be divided into three groups: the erector spinae, semispinalis, and deep posterior spinal group. As seen in figure 2.6, the erector spinae, the most powerful of the spinal extensors, is made up of three columns: the spinalis, longissimus, and iliocostalis. Deep to the erector spinae, the semispinalis is present only from the thoracic spine upward. Strengthening this muscle group can help prevent the common tendency for a slumped upper back posture. The deep posterior spinal group—interspinales, intertransversales, rotatores, and multifidus—is parallel in function to the transversus abdominis. Its primary role is stabilization of the spine and small movements of one vertebra relative to an adjacent vertebra (segmental movement). One of the members of this group, the multifidus (lumbar portion seen in figure 2.6), has been shown to be particularly vital for stabilization and rehabilitation of the spine. The multifidus spans more vertebrae and has the potential to produce more force than the other components of this deep group because of its attachments. Therefore, use of this muscle is often emphasized.

In terms of action, contraction of both sides of these three muscle groups (erector spinae, semispinalis, and deep posterior spinal group) produces spinal extension, whereas contraction of one side (except for the interspinales) can produce lateral flexion to the same side. Contraction of one side of the erector spinae (except for the spinalis) can also produce rotation to the same side, while contraction of one side of the semispinalis and some of the deep posterior spinal group (the multifidus and rotatores) can produce rotation to the opposite side. When you perform an exercise such as Back Extension Prone (page 66), both sides of the erector spinae, semispinalis, and

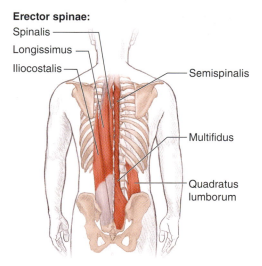

Erector spinae:
Spinalis
Longissimus
Iliocostalis
Semispinalis
Multifidus
Quadratus lumborum

Figure 2.6 Spinal extensors and the quadratus lumborum (back view of vertebral column). The three columns (spinalis, longissimus, and iliocostalis) of the erector spinae are shown on the left side. The semispinalis, multifidus (a key member of the deep posterior spinal group), and quadratus lumborum are shown on the right side of the spine.

deep posterior spinal group can produce the desired extension of the spine, with the erector spinae being the most powerful. However, when rotating to the right, such as in Swimming (page 184), two columns of the right erector spinae, the left semispinalis, the left multifidus, and the left rotatores primarily work to produce the desired spinal rotation while maintaining a lifted spine off the mat in extension.

Quadratus Lumborum and Iliopsoas

The quadratus lumborum and iliopsoas also have important actions relative to the spine that come into play with Pilates mat work. As shown in figure 2.6, the quadratus lumborum attaches from the pelvis to the sides of the lumbar spine and the lowest rib. When one side contracts, the quadratus lumborum can produce spinal lateral flexion to the same side.

The iliopsoas (figure 2.7a) is a powerful muscle that is primarily known for its ability to lift the leg high to the front (hip flexion), which will be discussed in the next chapter. As seen in figure 2.7b, its attachments onto the spine also allow the iliopsoas to serve a vital role in helping to maintain the desired normal curvature of the lumbar spine and assist with lateral flexion of the lumbar spine.

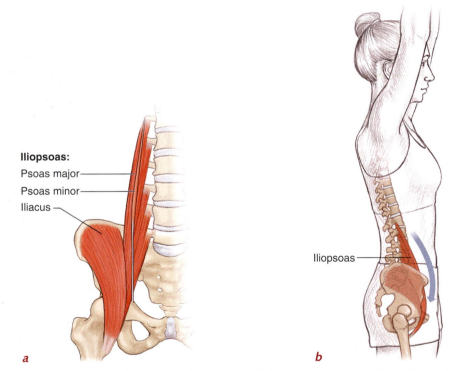

Iliopsoas:
Psoas major
Psoas minor
Iliacus

Iliopsoas

a   b

Figure 2.7   Iliopsoas muscle *(a)* primarily made up of the psoas major and iliacus (front view); *(b)* helping to maintain the lumbar curve (side view).

Use of Spinal Muscles in Pilates

Identifying the muscles actually used in a given Pilates mat exercise is often complicated by various factors. One important consideration is the relationship of the body to gravity throughout a given exercise. In addition, many Pilates movements utilize a simultaneous contraction of multiple spinal muscles in order to achieve the desired form and integration of the Pilates principles.

Influence of Gravity on Spinal Muscle Use

The position of the body relative to gravity greatly influences which muscles will work in a given mat exercise. When you are lying on your back and facing the ceiling (supine position), spinal flexion occurs against gravity and so provides a greater challenge for the abdominals. Therefore, many Pilates mat exercises that aim to improve abdominal strength and endurance incorporate a supine position, such as some of the exercises in chapter 5. To emphasize improving the muscular strength and endurance of the obliques, rotation can be added to spinal flexion performed from a supine position or lateral flexion performed from a side-lying position where it is effectively opposed by gravity, such as some exercises in chapter 8. Lateral flexion can also be produced by the quadratus lumborum and spinal extensors. Subtle changes in the alignment of the legs, pelvis, and spine influence the relative contributions of these muscles during exercises involving lateral flexion. From a prone position (lying on your belly, face toward the mat), spinal extension occurs against gravity and so provides a greater challenge for the spinal extensors. Many Pilates mat exercises that aim to improve muscular strength and endurance of the spinal extensors incorporate a prone position, such as some of the exercises in chapter 9.

Cocontraction of Spinal Muscles

Pilates often requires a skilled contraction of different spinal muscle groups at the same time, a process called *cocontraction*. Back Extension Prone (page 66) provides an example of cocontraction. Even though the spinal extensors are the muscles being focused on for strength, a cocontraction of the abdominals is used to limit the magnitude of hyperextension that occurs in the lower back and help protect the lower lumbar spine, which is very vulnerable to injury.

Some of the more complex mat exercises involve a changing of the body's position relative to gravity in different phases of the movement, necessitating a modification in how the spinal muscles work. An example is Jackknife (page 123), in which the abdominals are predominantly used to flex the spine for the rollover phase, but cocontraction of the spinal extensors becomes important in the phase when the legs and trunk reach up toward the ceiling. Cocontraction is widely used in Pilates both to help with the achievement of optimal technique and to reduce risk of injury for the back.

Discovering Your Powerhouse

The powerhouse, or core, can be described as the area from the bottom of the rib cage to a line across the hip joints in the front and to the base of the buttocks in the back. Joseph Pilates placed great emphasis on the powerhouse, considering it a physical center of the body from which all Pilates movements should proceed. Many Pilates exercises are designed to strengthen the powerhouse, and there is a desire to keep the powerhouse working consistently throughout a given exercise. If the powerhouse is being used appropriately, the limbs should be able to move in a more coordinated and connected manner.

Some Pilates practitioners and many people in disciplines such as dance, fitness, and rehabilitation also refer to this area as the *core* and the desired maintenance of appropriate positioning and activation during movement as *core stability*. Core stability can be thought of as the ability to keep the pelvis and spine in the desired position while moving the limbs or the whole body through space without undesired distortions or compensations. Someone who is not maintaining desired control of this area in a given movement and who arches the lower back or moves the pelvis excessively is often said to have a weak core or demonstrate poor core stability or poor core control.

In Pilates terminology, the powerhouse consists of the abdomen, lower back, and pelvis. The abdominals and the lower spinal extensors are considered particularly key to the concept of the powerhouse and have already been discussed earlier in this chapter. In addition, the concept of the powerhouse includes the pelvis and, in general, the primary muscles that influence the movement and stability of the pelvis.

Each hip bone (os coxae) is connected firmly in the back to one side of the sacrum at the paired sacroiliac joints. The hip bones are also connected to each other in the front via a joint called the pubic symphysis. These strong connections allow the hip bones along with the interposed sacrum and coccyx to act as a unit, referred to as the *pelvic girdle.* As described earlier in the chapter, each hip bone is actually made up of three bones—the ilium, ischium, and pubis. Each of these bones has landmarks commonly used for identifying body alignment.

Bony Landmarks of the Pelvis and Hip

Bones have distinct markings such as indentations, openings, lines, and protrusions that are collectively termed *bony landmarks.* The selected bony landmarks described here and shown in figure 2.8 are helpful in identifying core alignment and stability.

- **Iliac crest.** The ilium is the large upper winglike portion of the hip bone. If you move your hands down from your waist, you will feel a large ridge of bone. This is the upper border of the ilium. This convex border is called the *iliac crest.*

- **Anterior superior iliac spines (ASIS).** If you slide your hands to the front of the iliac crests and then slightly down, you will feel a bony prominence on each side of the front of the pelvis. These paired prominences are called the *anterior superior iliac spines (ASIS).*

- **Pubic symphysis (PS).** The pubis forms the lower and front portion of each hip bone. The pubis of each hip bone join at the front to form the pubic symphysis, connected by a disc of cartilage. You can see the pubic symphysis by standing with your side to a mirror. The pubic symphysis is the portion of the lower pelvis that is the most forward. It is abbreviated as *PS* in figure 2.8.

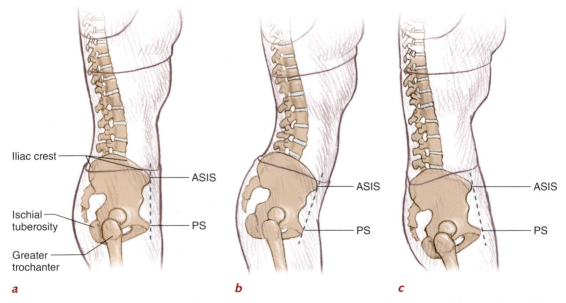

Figure 2.8   Bony landmarks and standing pelvic alignment (side view): *(a)* neutral pelvic alignment; *(b)* anterior pelvic tilt; *(c)* posterior pelvic tilt.

- **Ischial tuberosity.** The ischium is a very strong bone in the lower and back portion of each hip bone. The lowest portion of each ischium has a roughened prominence, the forward portion on which we sit, termed the *ischial tuberosity,* or *sit bone.* You can palpate these tuberosities easily while sitting on the floor. Lean forward and place your fingertips under the bottom of the pelvis from behind. Slowly begin to rock your weight back to sit upright. The tuberosities will press down against your fingers.

- **Greater trochanter.** The hip joint is formed between the hollowed socket of the pelvis (acetabulum) and the rounded top (head) of the femur. A large projection toward the top of the femur faces outward. This projection is called the *greater trochanter.* When you are standing, the tip of the greater trochanter is at about the same level as the center of the head of the femur as it sits in the hip joint. Although not a part of the pelvis, this landmark is included because a line between the right and left greater trochanters can be used to mark the lower border of the powerhouse. You can palpate the greater trochanter by placing your thumb on the side of the crest of the ilium and reaching down the side of the thigh with the middle finger. When you internally and externally rotate the leg, you should feel the greater trochanter move beneath the middle finger.

Movement and Alignment of the Pelvis

Learning to identify a neutral pelvic position, an anterior pelvic tilt, and a posterior pelvic tilt and to achieve the positions desired in a given Pilates exercise are important goals of Pilates. Because the pelvis moves primarily as a unit, the large movements of the pelvis mostly occur at the lumbosacral joint, the junction of the lower back with the pelvis. Stand upright with your side to a mirror to observe the first set of movements of the pelvis and related changes in the lumbar spine. Place one index finger on each ASIS to aid in seeing the desired relationships.

When in a *neutral pelvic alignment,* each ASIS (the top projections of the front of the pelvis) is aligned vertically with the pubic symphysis (the front of the lower pelvis). If a piece of poster board were held vertically from the pubic symphysis, both the right and left ASIS would touch this poster board (figure 2.8*a*). In this neutral position of the pelvis, the lumbar spine is also generally in a neutral position, exhibiting its natural curve, not a diminished or exaggerated curve.

In contrast, if you rotate the top of the pelvis forward, each ASIS will be in front of the pubic symphysis; this is logically termed an *anterior pelvic tilt* (figure 2.8*b*). This anterior movement of the pelvis will tend to increase the arch of the lumbar spine (extension or hyperextension). Check to see if you can see a change in your lower back curvature.

Conversely, if you rotate the top of the pelvis backward, each ASIS will be behind the pubic symphysis. This is a *posterior pelvic tilt* (figure 2.8*c*). With a posterior pelvic tilt, the curve of the lower back is decreased, flattened, or even reversed to round in the other direction, depending on the mobility of your spine.

Although these are the most emphasized aspects of pelvic movement, the pelvis can also move in other planes. The pelvis can tilt from side to side. When the right ASIS is lower than the left ASIS, this is called a right lateral tilt of the pelvis. Conversely, when the left ASIS is lower than the right ASIS, this is a left lateral tilt. This is observed more easily from a front view, such as facing a mirror. Lastly, the pelvis can rotate. When the right ASIS is in front of the left ASIS, this is left pelvic rotation. When the left ASIS is in front of the right ASIS, this is right pelvic rotation.

Although classically these movements of the pelvis are described in a standing position, they apply to many other positions used in Pilates, such as lying on the back, lying facedown, sitting, kneeling, or being supported on the hands and feet. In Pilates starting positions or exercises requiring a neutral pelvis, ideally the ASIS would be aligned with each other so they are level versus laterally tilted and square instead of rotated, as well as being in the same plane as the pubic symphysis.

Pelvic Muscles of the Powerhouse

Many of the muscles of the spine attach to the pelvis as well as the spine or rib cage. Although the customary actions of these muscles relative to the spine have already been described, there are times when these muscles act to move the pelvis in isolation or in conjunction with the spine. So when the rectus abdominis and obliques contract, they are capable of creating a posterior tilt of the pelvis as well as spinal flexion. The spinal extensors are capable of creating an anterior tilt of the pelvis as well as spinal extension. The iliopsoas is capable of creating an anterior tilt of the pelvis as well as extension of the lumbar spine. And the quadratus lumborum can produce a lateral tilt of the pelvis as well as lateral flexion of the spine. One of the benefits of the Pilates method is that it incorporates exercises that use the multiple potential actions of these important core muscles. For example, Chest Lift (page 54) uses the abdominals to flex the spine, whereas Pelvic Curl (page 52) emphasizes the use of the abdominals to create a posterior pelvic tilt.

In many instances, the potential actions of these pelvic muscles are used to prevent an undesired action and create core stability rather than actual visible movement. For example, when the iliopsoas contracts rigorously to support the weight of the legs in Hundred (page 78), the potential action of the abdominals to create a posterior tilt is used to prevent the undesired anterior tilt associated with the iliopsoas so that the pelvis can remain stable and protect the lower back. Another example is when the quadratus lumborum works in a postural manner to help determine the distance between the top of the pelvis and the rib cage, a function used frequently in Pilates to keep the pelvis level.

Many other muscles that attach to the pelvis are known more for their actions of moving the legs at the hip joint than moving the pelvis. However, two muscle groups that are commonly included in a discussion of the powerhouse, or core, are the gluteus maximus and pelvic floor muscles.

The *gluteus maximus* is a powerful muscle that is pulled into play with movements such as jumping, cycling, stair climbing, and uphill running. In these activities, the muscle works as an extensor of the hip (to be described in chapter 3), but it can also function in a postural role to create a posterior pelvic tilt and help maintain core stability. The original Pilates work emphasized gripping this muscle and encouraged squeezing the buttocks together as if to pinch a dime between them. This approach may have been adopted because of the common tendency to lose tone in these muscles with aging. As they age, people often give up the powerful activities that effectively challenge the gluteus maximus. While still acknowledging the importance of strengthening this muscle, many current schools of Pilates put less emphasis on continuously gripping the gluteus maximus throughout a given Pilates exercise in favor of strategies of stabilization that are more functional in regard to everyday activities. Examples of alternative strategies include emphasizing a less forceful or continuous contraction of the gluteus maximus as well as combining its use with other core muscles such as the abdominals.

The *pelvic floor muscles,* consisting of the levator ani and coccygeus as shown in figure 2.9, form the funnel-shaped floor of the pelvic cavity. This muscular sling stretches between the coccyx and the front of the pelvis as well as between the lateral walls of the pelvis. The pelvic floor muscles provide support for the terminal part of the rectum, the prostate, and the urethra in males and the rectum, the vagina, and the urethra in females. Balanced strength and activation of the pelvic floor muscles is considered by some to be another important element of core stability. Simultaneous contraction of the diaphragm and pelvic floor muscles will help maintain the abdominal contents within the abdominopelvic cavity, while the transversus abdominis functions to enhance stabilization of the spine. Research indicates a close association between the pelvic floor muscles and transversus abdominis and that contraction of the pelvic floor muscles can be used to facilitate contraction of the transversus abdominis, and vice versa. Adequate strength of the pelvic floor muscles may also be helpful in preventing some types of urinary incontinence. Almost one-quarter of adult women in the United States are affected by pelvic floor disorders, and many studies focus on women (Kincade et al. 2007). However, pelvic floor exercises for men before prostate surgery may aid with urinary continence after surgery.

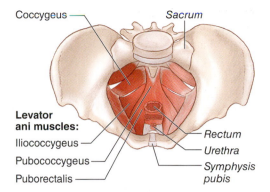

Figure 2.9 View of pelvic floor from above showing the three parts of the levator ani—the pubococcygeus, puborectalis, and iliococcygeus—and the coccygeus muscles.

Although use of the pelvic floor muscles was not specifically emphasized in the original work of Joseph Pilates, some current schools of Pilates have integrated targeting the pelvic floor muscles into their approach. One of the recommended protocols in the medical community (Kincade et al. 2005) is to perform a 10-second contraction while gently exhaling with the mouth open, followed by 10 seconds of relaxation, for 15 repetitions, three times per day. For women, beginning by tightening the pelvic floor muscles as if to prevent passing gas, then bringing the tightening movement forward to the muscles around the vagina, and lastly thinking of drawing the vaginal contraction upward toward the small of the back can be helpful for desired activation of the pelvic floor muscles. In Pilates mat work, the pelvic floor is often less formally addressed by encouraging both men and women to pull the pelvic floor muscles inward and upward while activating the transversus abdominis before and during the execution of many exercises. Optimal pelvic floor activation and function is still an area of controversy.

Full-Body Alignment Basics

Pelvic alignment has been discussed already, and a similar naming of positions and analysis of muscles that affect alignment of a given region could be done for most segments of the body. In this section, we will focus on selected areas that are particularly key in Pilates. Optimal positioning of these body segments often involves a relationship in which healthy joint mechanics is encouraged and excessive use of muscles or excess stress to joints is prevented. Realize that alignment problems can have many causes, and although some common suggestions for improvement are provided, it is vital to check with your physician to see if these recommendations are appropriate for you. This will help to rule out causes other than strength and flexibility imbalances or suboptimal patterns of activating the associated muscles.

Standing Alignment

Ideal standing alignment is a position in which the head, torso, and pelvis are aligned above one another and above the feet so that very little muscle activity is required to maintain their position.

Practically, this concept can be reflected by viewing the body from the side and noting the positioning of surface landmarks relative to a plumb line, a suspended cord with a weight attached to the bottom that provides an absolute vertical line. Other vertical lines such as a vertical seam in a mirror can also serve this function. Stand with your side to the plumb line or vertical line so that the lower end of the line falls just in front of your ankle. With ideal standing postural alignment, the following external landmarks would be located right along this vertical line (as seen in figure 2.10a):

- Earlobe
- Middle of the tip of the shoulder
- Middle of the rib cage
- Greater trochanter (projection on lateral femur)
- The area just in front of the middle of the knee
- The area just in front of the ankle

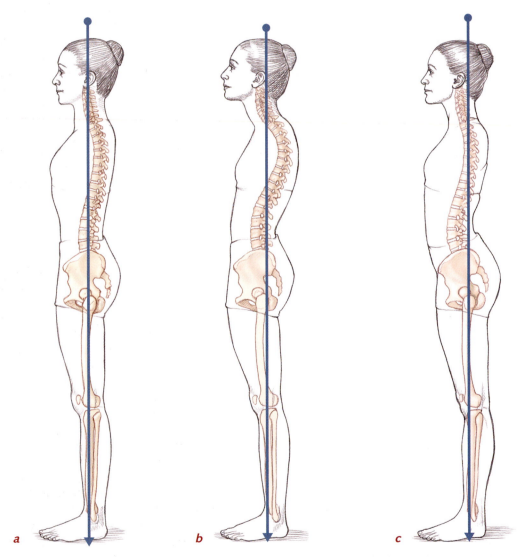

Figure 2.10　Ideal standing alignment and common deviations (side view): *(a)* ideal standing alignment with plumb line; *(b)* cervical lordosis and kyphosis; *(c)* lumbar lordosis.

Although not always the case, optimal positioning of these landmarks ideally represents a situation where the following underlying alignment goals also are met:

- Feet neutral, not rolled in (pronated) or out (supinated)
- Knees straight but not straightened so far they bow backward (knee hyperextension)
- Pelvis neutral, not anteriorly or posteriorly tilted
- Spine with normal curve, not decreased or increased
- Scapulae neutral and shoulders open, not rolled forward
- Head above shoulders, not jutting forward

Common Spinal Alignment Deviations

One common source of alignment problems is an exaggeration of the curvature in a given region of the spine. Exaggeration of the cervical curve (cervical lordosis) is often associated with the alignment problem called *forward head,* in which the chin juts forward and the earlobe is forward relative to the plumb line and shoulders (figure 2.10*b*). An increased curve in the thoracic region, termed *kyphosis,* is particularly common with aging. Increasing strength and the use of the upper spinal extensors often can improve this condition, at least in its earlier stages. Lumbar lordosis or lumbar hyperlordosis refers to an increased curve in the lower back region, commonly accompanied by an anterior pelvic tilt (figure 2.10*c*). This common postural problem, which may increase the risk of lower back issues, often can be helped by developing greater strength and use of the abdominals as well as adequate flexibility of the lower spinal extensors and iliopsoas.

When addressing these common spinal alignment deviations, it is important to realize that the goal is to not overcorrect and remove the normal curves of the spine. Such an action would create another spinal problem in which the lumbar and sometimes other curvatures actually are below normal in terms of magnitude. This condition is termed *flat back posture* and is theorized to interfere with optimal functioning of the spine.

Scapular Movements and Alignment Deviations

The shoulder girdle is composed of one clavicle and one scapula. Unlike the pelvic girdle, which is firmly attached to the spine via the sacroiliac joints, the scapula slides on the rib cage, with only muscles connecting it to the spine. The only true bony connection of the shoulder girdle to the axial skeleton is the sternoclavicular joint, the small joint between the clavicle and the sternum. Because of these limited connections, movements of the shoulder girdle are very dependent on muscles, and muscle imbalances can easily lead to alignment problems. Movements of the shoulder girdle can be simplified by referring to the movements of the scapula, which are shown in figure 2.11 on page 24.

Scapular elevation involves lifting the scapula up toward your ear; scapular depression means bringing it down toward your waist (figure 2.11*a*). In scapular abduction, the scapula is moved farther away from the spine, while in scapular adduction it is brought closer toward the spine (figure 2.11*b*). In upward rotation, the scapula is rotated so the upper outer portion moves upward; downward rotation involves the opposite motion (figure 2.11*c*).

When the arm moves, ideally the scapula moves in a coordinated manner that allows the upper humerus (head) to maintain proper positioning in the shoulder socket (glenoid fossa) located on the scapula. One of the most common alignment problems in this region is related to raising the arm to the side or front. This movement is accompanied naturally by a smooth upward rotation of the scapula, but many people add undesired excessive elevation of the scapula. This tendency can be countered by coordinated use of the muscles that depress the scapula, the serratus anterior and lower trapezius (shown in figure 2.12 on page 24).

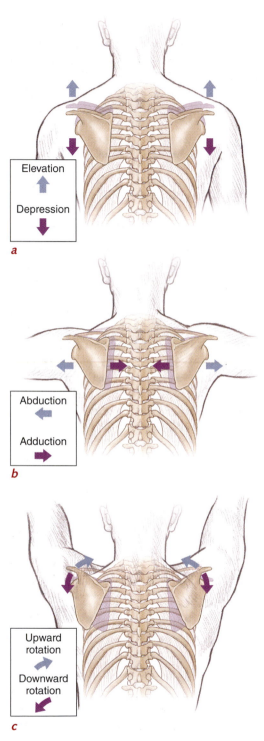

a

Elevation

Depression

b

Abduction

Adduction

c

Upward
rotation

Downward
rotation

Figure 2.11 Movements of the scapulae (back view of trunk): *(a)* elevation and depression; *(b)* abduction and adduction; *(c)* upward rotation and downward rotation.

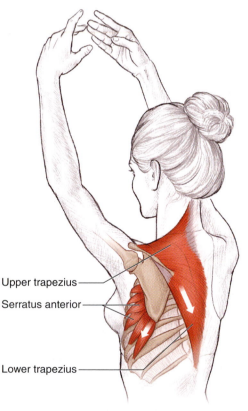

Upper trapezius

Serratus anterior

Lower trapezius

Figure 2.12 Use of the scapular depressors (serratus anterior and lower trapezius) to prevent excessive elevation of each scapula as the arms are raised overhead.

As with the pelvis, in many instances the function of the scapular muscles may be related more to posture or prevention of an undesired scapular motion so that stability is maintained than to producing visible movement. An example of the former is rolled shoulders. In this posture, the shoulders round forward and the scapulae separate excessively. Often this can be helped by developing greater strength and use of the scapular adductors, including the trapezius. The latter function of stability is operative in many Pilates exercises in which the body weight is supported by the arms. For example, when lifting the pelvis off the mat from a sitting position (Back Support, page 138), gravity tends to make the scapulae elevate markedly. Forceful contraction of the scapular depressors, including the serratus anterior and lower trapezius, is necessary to keep the scapulae in their desired neutral position, protect the shoulders from injury, and allow the shoulder muscles to perform their desired function.

Putting Alignment Into Action in Pilates Mat Work

Many of the Pilates exercises in this book are designed to strengthen muscles that are important for alignment and core stability. However, strength alone will not necessarily create the desired results. It also is important to learn to feel correct alignment and core stability, to hone skills for quickly achieving this alignment, and to practice utilizing this alignment in the exercises in this book as well as during other appropriate activities in your life. Research suggests that with repetitive activation of the desired muscles in the appropriate manner, over time your body will automatically start utilizing these more optimal strategies.

Many common cues are used with Pilates to try to achieve the desired static or dynamic alignment in a given exercise. These cues, or directives, offer practical ways to help you apply many of the principles discussed in chapter 1 and in this chapter. Some cues used with the exercises in this book are described in this section. Others are described in the chapter introductions or with the specific exercises in chapters 4 through 9. In the original Pilates approach, many of these cues were exaggerated. However, the desire to create strategies that are more similar to those needed in functional movements has led various current approaches to apply some of these cues in a modified or less rigorous manner. This functional emphasis also led to the development of additional cues to encourage a neutral position of the pelvis or spine in appropriate exercises.

- **Draw the navel or abdominal wall to the spine, or scoop.** These cues are designed to counter the common error of having the abdominal wall bulge outward when the abdominals are activated and to encourage a flattening or pulling inward of the abdomen. With the first cue you can imagine that a string is attached to the inside of the navel, with the string tightening to pull the navel toward the front of your spine. Drawing the abdominal wall inward toward the spine can be likened to tightening a corset such that the circumference of your waist feels smaller. It can also be thought of as scooping or hollowing the abdominal area inward. If you have difficulty finding this muscular control, place the palm of one hand on your lower abdomen, and press the wall outward into your hand to feel the undesired position; then try to draw the abdominal wall inward so your hand lowers. Think of the hand pressing flat toward the spine or the hand scooping the abdomen, as if making a hollow in the sand at the beach. The cue of drawing the abdominal wall inward has been shown to be effective in recruiting the deep transversus abdominis as well as achieving the aesthetic goal of a flatter abdomen.

- **Bring the spine to the mat.** When lying on your back, firmly draw the abdominal wall inward to bring the lumbar spine closer toward or in touch with the mat, depending on your natural curve and flexibility. The change in the contact of the spine with the mat can be used to help maintain and monitor core stability. For example, when the legs are held off the mat in exercises such as Hundred (page 78), inadequate abdominal stabilization would cause an anterior tilt of the pelvis and arching of the lower back, lifting the lower back off the mat and potentially injuring the lower spine. So in exercises like this, the cue is often given to keep the legs at a height (the closer to vertical, the easier the exercise) at which the lower spine can remain close to or in touch with the mat, with the pelvis totally stationary. This directive involves an intentional decrease in the natural lumbar curve and, generally, a slight posterior tilt of the pelvis to help prevent lumbar hyperextension.

• **Pull up with the abdominals.** Pulling the lower attachment of the abdominals (rectus abdominis and obliques) upward can produce a posterior pelvic tilt. Often this cue is used to encourage creation of a posterior pelvic tilt and flexion of the lumbar spine in exercises that require this full rounding, such as Rolling Back (page 100). The cue is also used to prevent or limit an anterior pelvic tilt in exercises in which the limbs are moving or the back is arching, such as Double Kick (page 181).

• **Keep the rib cage down and back.** When trying to stabilize the trunk, a common mistake is to contract the spinal extensors so the rib cage juts forward (rib-leading). The upper attachment of the abdominals onto the rib cage can pull the front of the rib cage slightly down and back to prevent this undesired rib-leading and hold the rib cage in its desired neutral alignment in many exercises. In other exercises involving spinal flexion, pulling the front of the lower rib cage down and back can aid in getting the desired maximum spinal flexion to help with achieving a full C curve.

• **Make a C curve.** A common error when flexing the spine is to flex only the neck and the upper thoracic spine while leaving the rest of the spine flat or hyperextended. Another frequent problem is to have most of the curve occur in the thoracic spine, a region of the spine that is naturally concave to the front but is already excessively rounded (kyphosis) in static alignment in many people. Instead, the intent of this cue is to include flexion of the lumbar spine—a region naturally concave to the back and often tight, making flexion in this area more challenging. This will aid with distributing the forward curvature as much as possible throughout the spine while pulling in the abdominal wall so the head, spine, and pelvis form a C shape that is concave to the front.

• **Lengthen your neck.** A common alignment problem is an excessive arch in the neck so that the chin projects forward in static alignment (forward head posture) or during movement. Thinking of lengthening or stretching the back of the neck can help counter this tendency. For example, when lying on your back, bring your chin slightly down and back while rotating your head slightly forward so that the contact of the back of the head with the mat moves down toward the base of the skull. Anatomically, this involves using the neck flexors while focusing on relaxing often excessively tight neck extensors.

• **Bring your chin to your chest.** The cue to lengthen the neck is also linked with the cue to bring the chin to the chest. In original Pilates work, the cue to flex the neck so that the chin comes toward the sternum while the back of the neck lengthens was often exaggerated in many exercises involving spinal flexion. Bringing the head closer to the chest can help with the desired emphasis on greater use of the abdominals while producing less stress on some of the neck muscles in many supine abdominal exercises. However, many current approaches encourage a moderate use of this cue so that the head is in line with an arc created by the thoracic spine (a small fist or lemon could fit between the chin and chest).

• **Move one vertebra at a time, or use a smooth sequential movement of each vertebra.** A common error is to have a large chunk of the spine move as a solid unit, often causing jerky movements or making a portion of the spine appear flat rather than arched or curved.

In contrast, the desire is precise consecutive movement of one vertebra relative to the next vertebra, aimed at achieving full movement in each segment of the spine that is involved in the exercise. For example, during the up phase of Roll-Up (page 73), the vertebrae should lift one at a time off the mat from top to bottom and lower sequentially in the reverse order on the down phase.

- **Keep a neutral pelvis and lumbar spine.** Most of the previous cues encourage flexion of the spine, often accompanied by a posterior pelvic tilt. However, some current approaches hold that too much emphasis on flexion may not be desirable. They encourage training multiple core muscles to cocontract to maintain the natural curves of the spine, believing this will aid in creating a stable spine in many everyday movements that do not incorporate spinal flexion. Practically, if neutral positioning is the goal, a coordinated contraction of the abdominals and spinal extensors is often required to allow the natural lumbar curvature to remain and the ASIS and pubic symphysis to be in a neutral relationship. For example, when lying on your back, think about drawing in the abdominal wall gently while reaching the sit bones away from the rib cage to encourage this cocontraction and limit the tendency to posteriorly tilt the pelvis or flatten the lumbar spine. In some exercises, cocontraction of the hip flexors and abdominals is another strategy for achieving or maintaining a neutral pelvis. Some approaches to Pilates also encourage maintaining a neutral pelvis in some exercises that involve flexion of the upper spine, such as Chest Lift (page 54). This can be helpful for learning more isolated control and awareness of the neutral pelvis. However, exercises that involve marked flexion of the lumbar spine, such as Roll-Up (page 73) naturally tend to be accompanied by a posterior pelvic tilt, and trying to maintain a neutral pelvis can place excess stress on the lower back.

- **Sit tall.** A common alignment error in sitting is to let the spine collapse downward, with the lumbar spine going into flexion and the pelvis posteriorly tilting. Think of lifting the upper back and the area of the head just behind the ears toward the ceiling, with the weight of the trunk right over the sit bones. Anatomically, slight use of the upper back extensors balanced with the abdominals can produce the desired lift in the thoracic spine without rib-leading. Another desired strategy, similar to that described in the last section, is to think of pulling the lower region of the abdominals slightly in and up to foster use of the transversus abdominis while simultaneously lifting the center of the back of the pelvis upward to encourage use of the multifidus. This cocontraction provides deep segmental support to the lower spine and encourages the maintenance of some of the natural lumbar curve. Activation of the iliopsoas can also be used to help maintain some of the natural lumbar curve as well as keep the upper trunk from falling back. Shifting the pelvis forward (hip flexion) while thinking of lifting the inside of the pelvis upward may help promote iliopsoas activation.

- **Maintain a flat back.** The term *flat back* refers to a position in which the trunk is approximately straight when viewed from the side; the side of the shoulder, rib cage, and pelvis are in line. This term can be used to describe the trunk in various positions including kneeling, being supported on the hands and feet, or sitting. The term is not literal—the spine still maintains its natural curvatures, but there is a feeling of being elongated as just described with sitting tall. Achievement of this flat back position involves a skillful simultaneous contraction of the abdominals and spinal extensors.

- **Keep the scapulae down to neutral.** This cue can be used to prevent the common alignment error of having the shoulders lift up toward the ears as the arms move. Anatomically, think of using the scapular depressors to pull the scapulae slightly downward before lifting the arms to encourage use of these muscles as the arms move. However, the goal is not to hold the scapulae excessively downward or in place but rather to help establish a neutral position of the scapulae as they naturally rotate upward. This is achieved with a balance of use between the upper trapezius, which elevates the scapulae, and the lower trapezius, which depresses the scapulae, as shown in figure 2.12 (page 24). You can also focus on keeping distance between the shoulders and the ears by using a less forceful contraction of the upper trapezius to prevent excessive undesired elevation of the scapulae with overhead movement of the arms.

• **Stretch or reach your arms and legs.** The cue of reaching the limbs outward is used to achieve the desired long line and dynamic of many Pilates exercises. Anatomically the joints of the limbs are in a straight line rather than bent or hyperextended. When the body is straight with arms overhead and legs elongated, such as the beginning position of Roll-Up (page 73), imagine someone gently pulling on your fingertips while someone else gently pulls on your toes in the opposite direction as you maintain strong core stability.

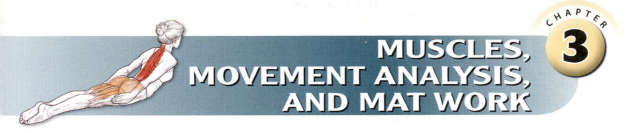
MUSCLES, MOVEMENT ANALYSIS, AND MAT WORK

Understanding the muscles that are working in a given mat exercise will help you apply the Pilates foundation principles discussed in chapter 1 and the alignment principles discussed in chapter 2. While chapter 2 focused on the spine, this chapter will add the movements and muscles of the major joints of the upper and lower extremities. We will describe the principles of how muscles work to produce isolated and complex full-body movements and present a simple schema that can be used to analyze the mat exercises. The chapter concludes with an explanation of the format used to describe the mat exercises and summary recommendations for beginning the mat work.

Joints and Their Movements

The bones described in chapter 2 (figure 2.1, page 10) connect to form joints. The way bones connect and the shapes of the surfaces that come together are used to classify joints into specific types. Different types of joints have different movement potential, and standardized terminology is used to describe the movements that are possible at a given joint.

Types of Joints

There are three major types of joints: fibrous, cartilaginous, and synovial. With fibrous joints, the adjacent bones are directly linked with fibrous tissue, such as the sutures of the skull. With cartilaginous joints, the adjacent bones are directly linked with cartilage, such as occurs in the spine, where the bodies of adjacent vertebrae are connected with an intervertebral disc as shown in figure 2.3, page 12. In contrast to fibrous and cartilaginous joints, synovial joints actually have a small space between the adjacent bones, called a *joint cavity,* that contains synovial fluid. Synovial fluid has a consistency similar to egg white and is important for joint lubrication. With synovial joints, the adjacent bones are connected indirectly with a sleevelike structure of fibrous tissue (the joint capsule) and strong bands of fibrous tissue (the ligaments).

Synovial joints are particularly important for large body movements. Synovial joints can be further subdivided into six types, named according to their shape. Two of these types of synovial joints—ball-and-socket and hinge joints—are particularly key for understanding limb movements. A ball-and-socket joint is formed from the rounded head of one bone and the concave cup, or socket, in the adjoining bone. Ball-and-socket joints are the most freely movable type of joint in the body, and they appear at the roots of the limbs—the shoulder and hip joints. With a hinge joint, a spool-shaped surface fits into a concave surface. The elbow, knee, and ankle are all classified as hinge joints.

Anatomical Position and Joint Movement Terminology

Standardized terminology has been developed to describe movements of synovial joints. This terminology is vital for analyzing movement and predicting the muscles that are important for producing a given movement. These basic joint movements are defined in reference to anatomical position.

In anatomical position (figure 3.1) a person is standing upright with the feet together or slightly separated, toes pointing forward. The arms are down by the sides with the palms facing forward. This is considered the beginning position or the zero position in terms of movement. A position in which the arm is down by the side would be considered zero degrees; if the arm is raised forward to shoulder height, this would be considered 90 degrees of flexion.

From anatomical position, there are six basic movements, some or all of which can occur at most synovial joints. These six basic joint movements can be grouped into three pairs of movement: flexion–extension (figure 3.2a and b), abduction–adduction (figure 3.2c), and external rotation–internal rotation (figure 3.2d). The components of each movement pair involve movement in the same plane but in the opposite direction.

In addition to these basic movements, specialized joint movements may occur. These movements are not adequately covered by use of the basic joint movement terminology. The specialized movements of the spine, pelvis, and scapula have already been described in chapter 2. Two other specialized joint movement pairs used in this book (shoulder horizontal abduction–horizontal adduction and ankle–foot plantar flexion–dorsiflexion) are described under the related basic movement descriptions that follow.

Figure 3.1 Anatomical position.

Flexion and Extension

Flexion refers to bending a joint by bringing the front surfaces of adjacent body parts together, such as when flexing the elbow, or in the case of the knee, bringing the back surfaces of adjacent body parts together. *Extension* refers to straightening the joint by bringing these adjacent body parts away from each other back toward anatomical position, such as when extending the elbow or knee, or beyond. A joint that moves in the direction of extension but beyond anatomical position is in *hyperextension*. Flexion and extension occur in a forward or backward direction relative to anatomical position. Related specialized terminology is used at the ankle, where *dorsiflexion* refers to flexing the foot by bringing the top, or dorsal, surface of the foot up toward the shin. *Ankle–foot plantar flexion* refers to pointing the foot by bringing the bottom, or plantar, surface of the foot down and away from the shin. These movements can be seen in figure 3.2a and b.

Abduction and Adduction

Abduction refers to movement away from the midline of the body such as when raising the arm (shoulder abduction) or leg (hip abduction) to the side. *Adduction* refers to the reverse movement of returning from a position of abduction back toward anatomical position. To help you remember these terms, remember that to abduct someone is to take that person away, whereas with adduction you are adding the part back in toward the midline to recreate anatomical position. These movements can be seen in figure 3.2c. Because the spine is located on the midline of the body, the specialized terminology of right lateral flexion and left lateral flexion has to be used to describe similar movements for the spine (previously shown in figure 2.4, page 13).

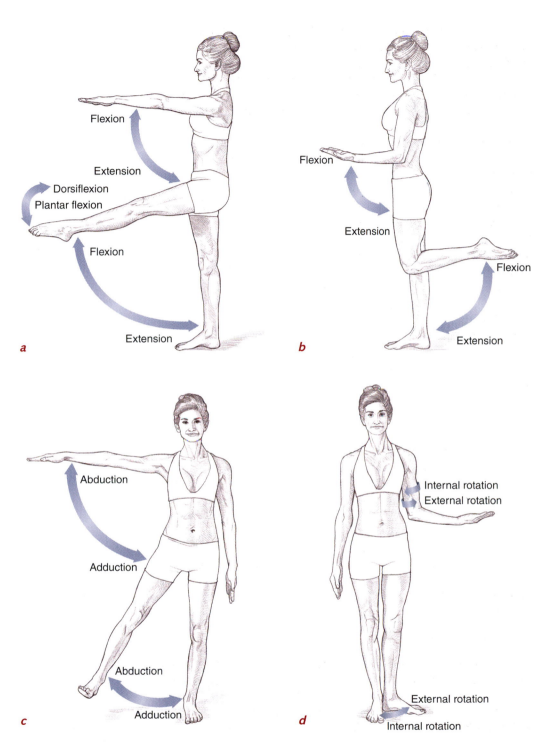

Figure 3.2 Major joint movements of the limbs: *(a)* shoulder and hip flexion–extension and ankle–foot plantar flexion–dorsiflexion; *(b)* elbow and knee flexion–extension; *(c)* shoulder and hip abduction–adduction; *(d)* shoulder and hip external rotation–internal rotation.

External and Internal Rotation

Rotation can be thought of as twisting around the length (longitudinal or vertical axis) of a limb or the spine. External or lateral rotation refers to moving the front surface of a limb outward or away from the midline of the body, such as when turning out the leg at the hip (hip external rotation). Internal or medial rotation refers to the opposite motion of bringing the front surface of a limb inward or toward the midline of the body from a position of external rotation or from anatomical position. These movements can be seen in figure 3.2d. Because the spine is located on the midline of the body, the specialized terminology of right rotation and left rotation has to be used to describe similar movements for the spine (previously shown in figure 2.4, page 13). From anatomical position, all these motions can be thought of as twisting motions around a vertical axis.

A related specialized movement pair that does not fit precisely into one category is shoulder horizontal abduction–horizontal adduction. In contrast to the other movements just described, this motion does not occur from pure anatomical position, but rather with the arm at shoulder height. However, in this case the arm moves horizontally relative to the floor. When moving away from the midline of the body, this movement is termed *shoulder horizontal abduction;* when moving toward the midline, it is *shoulder horizontal adduction.* The terminology of horizontal abduction and horizontal adduction can also be used for the hip joint when the thigh is moving horizontally and in line with the hip joint.

Muscles and Their Movements

Muscle cells are the only cells that have the ability to produce active tension and contract. Contractility is the ability of a muscle to shorten. There are three types of muscle tissue—smooth, cardiac, and skeletal—but for our discussion of Pilates, we will address only skeletal muscle tissue. As the name suggests, skeletal muscle attaches to bones and gives rise to movements at joints. Toward the end of a muscle, the contractile muscle cells end, but their connective tissue continues to attach directly or indirectly to the bone. The two types of indirect connections are a sheet of connective tissue called an *aponeurosis* and, most commonly, a cordlike structure of connective tissue called a *tendon.*

You can deduce the actions of a muscle at the interposed joint by looking at the location of a muscle and imagining one attachment of the muscle onto one bone being pulled toward the attachment of the same muscle onto a different bone. Using this deduction also reveals some common trends that will help you learn the actions of muscles that have similar locations. For example, for the hip, spine, elbow, and large muscles of the shoulder, those muscles located on the front of the body generally produce flexion and those on the back of the body extension. For the hip and shoulder, those muscles on the side of the body have an action of abduction. For the hip, muscles located toward the inside or midline of the body produce adduction. Muscles that are in between in their location often share the functions of both locations. For example, the tensor fasciae latae is located between the front and side of the hip joint and can produce both hip flexion and abduction. The knee bends in the opposite direction of these joints, and so the muscles exhibit an opposite relationship, with the extensors being located on the front and the flexors on the back of the body. Many of these muscles have additional actions, but their location will at least give you one of their primary actions.

For purposes of simplicity and clarity, the regional descriptions that follow are focused to include the most important muscles of major joints that also will be used in the description of Pilates mat work in chapters 4 through 9. The table for each region organizes muscles relative to production of a given movement. Tables include both primary and secondary muscles for most movements. The term *primary muscle* is used for a muscle that is particularly important or effective in producing the given movement. In contrast, a *secondary muscle* is a muscle that is not capable of producing as much force for the desired movement or is called into play in specialized situations such as in certain positions of the joint when high speed is required or when large forces are needed.

Muscles of the Spine

The major joints and muscles of the spine are described and illustrated in chapter 2. Table 3.1 provides a summary of the movements of the spine and the muscles that can produce them.

Table 3.1   Spinal Movements and Muscles

Joint movement	Primary muscles	Secondary muscles
Spinal flexion	Rectus abdominis External obliques Internal obliques	Iliopsoas (in select circumstances)
Spinal extension	Erector spinae: spinalis, longissimus, iliocostalis	Semispinalis Deep posterior spinal group: interspinales, intertransversales, rotatores, multifidus
Spinal lateral flexion	External oblique (same side) Internal oblique (same side) Quadratus lumborum (same side) Erector spinae (same side): spinalis, longissimus, iliocostalis	Semispinalis (same side) Deep posterior spinal group (same side): intertransversales, rotatores, multifidus Rectus abdominis (same side) Iliopsoas (lumbar region) (same side)
Spinal rotation	External oblique (opposite side) Internal oblique (same side) Erector spinae (same side): longissimus, iliocostalis	Semispinalis (opposite side) Deep posterior spinal group (opposite side): rotatores, multifidus

Muscles of the Lower Extremities

Table 3.2 (page 34) summarizes the movements of the major joints of the lower extremities and lists the muscles that produce them, and figure 3.3 (page 35) illustrates these muscles.

The hip joint is a ball-and-socket joint that allows all three movement pairs—flexion–extension, abduction–adduction, and external rotation–internal rotation. Beginning at the front of the hip, the rectus femoris and deeply located iliopsoas are ideally located for their function as the primary hip flexors.

The group of muscles in the inner thighs—the pectineus, adductor longus, adductor brevis, adductor magnus, and gracilis—is collectively referred to as the hip adductors. All these muscles, except for the adductor magnus, can also assist with hip flexion. The adductor magnus is the deepest muscle of this group. Because of its attachment running back toward the ischial tuberosities, its lower fibers assist with hip extension rather than flexion.

Table 3.2   Major Lower-Extremity Joint Movements and Muscles

Joint movement	Primary muscles	Secondary muscles
Hip flexion	Iliopsoas Rectus femoris	Sartorius Tensor fasciae latae Pectineus Adductor longus and brevis (lower ranges) Gracilis
Hip extension	Gluteus maximus Hamstrings: semitendinosus, semimembranosus, biceps femoris	Adductor magnus (lower fibers)
Hip abduction	Gluteus medius Gluteus minimus	Tensor fasciae latae Sartorius Iliopsoas (upper ranges)
Hip adduction	Adductor longus Adductor brevis Adductor magnus Gracilis	Pectineus
Hip external rotation	Gluteus maximus Deep outward rotators: piriformis, obturator internus, obturator externus, gemellus inferior, gemellus superior, quadratus femoris	Sartorius Biceps femoris
Hip internal rotation	Gluteus medius (anterior fibers) Gluteus minimus (anterior fibers)	Tensor fasciae latae Hamstrings: semitendinosus, semimembranosus
Knee flexion	Hamstrings: semitendinosus, semimembranosus, biceps femoris	Popliteus Gracilis Sartorius Gastrocnemius
Knee extension	Quadriceps femoris: rectus femoris, vastus medialis, vastus intermedius, vastus lateralis	Tensor fasciae latae (upper ranges)
Ankle–foot dorsiflexion	Tibialis anterior Extensor digitorum longus	Extensor hallucis longus Peroneus tertius
Ankle–foot plantar flexion	Gastrocnemius Soleus	Tibialis posterior Flexor hallucis longus Flexor digitorum longus Peroneus longus Peroneus brevis

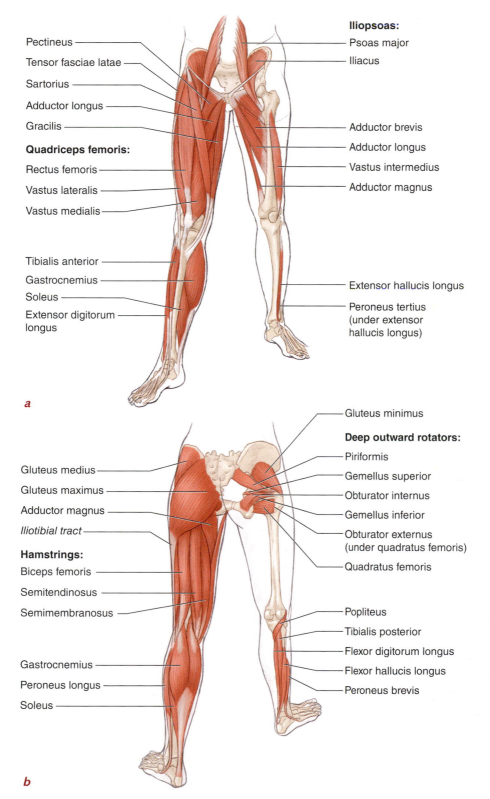

Figure 3.3 Major muscles of the lower extremities: (a) front view; (b) back view. Deeper muscles are shown on the left side of the body in figure a and on the right side of the body in figure b.

If you look toward the outside of the hip, the sartorius is the long, straplike muscle that runs diagonally across the front of the thigh to attach below the knee. It performs the actions of hip flexion, hip abduction, and hip external rotation. The tensor fasciae latae is located slightly more toward the outside of the thigh, and its actions are hip flexion, hip abduction, and hip internal rotation.

From a back view of the hip, the gluteal muscles are apparent. The location of the gluteus medius and gluteus minimus on the outside of the hip allows them to act as the primary abductors of the hip, while their front fibers are also capable of producing hip internal rotation. The large gluteus maximus, located more toward the back of the buttock, is a powerful extensor and external rotator of the hip. Deep to the gluteus maximus is a group of six small muscles, the deep outward rotators, that span between the pelvis and the greater trochanter of the femur. They are ideally located to act as external rotators of the hip.

The hamstrings (semitendinosus, semimembranosus, and biceps femoris) run down the back of the thigh and are hip extensors as well as knee flexors. The hamstring located more toward the outside, the biceps femoris, can also assist with hip external rotation when the knee is straight. The two hamstrings located more toward the inside, the semitendinosus and semimembranosus, can help with hip internal rotation.

The knee is classified as a modified hinge joint that primarily allows flexion and extension. The hamstrings function as the primary flexors of the knee, while the quadriceps femoris is the primary extensor. The quadriceps femoris forms much of the muscle mass of the front of the thigh and is made up of the rectus femoris and the three vastii (the vastus medialis, vastus intermedius, and vastus lateralis). Only the rectus femoris crosses the hip joint, which gives it the additional function of hip flexion as well as knee extension. Some muscles with primary actions at the hip and ankle joints also cross the knee and can assist with movements of the knee. In addition, a small muscle that is located deep and on the back side of the leg—the popliteus—also assists with flexing the knee and provides important stability for the knee during deep flexion and walking.

The ankle is a hinge joint with the movements of plantar flexion and dorsiflexion. The tibialis anterior and extensor digitorum longus on the front of the lower leg are the primary dorsiflexors of the ankle and foot. Their action of dorsiflexion can be assisted by two other muscles that cross the front of the ankle, the extensor hallucis longus and peroneus tertius. The calf muscles are the double-bellied gastrocnemius and the deeper and flatter muscle called the soleus. These muscles are the primary plantar flexors of the ankle and foot. Plantar flexion can also be assisted by two muscles running along the outside of the ankle, the peroneus longus and peroneus brevis, and three muscles that traverse along the inside of the ankle, the tibialis posterior, flexor hallucis longus, and flexor digitorum longus.

Muscles of the Upper Extremities

Table 3.3 summarizes the movements of major joints of the upper extremities and lists the muscles that can produce them, and figure 3.4 (page 38) illustrates these muscles.

The shoulder joint is a ball-and-socket joint that permits all three movement pairs—flexion–extension, abduction–adduction, and external rotation–internal rotation. The muscles primarily responsible for the large movements of the shoulder include the pectoralis major, the large chest muscle; the deltoid, the muscle that forms the rounded contour of the shoulder; and the latissimus dorsi, the very broad shoulder muscle located on the back of the body, with the help of the teres major.

Starting with the front view of the body, the anterior deltoid and the upper (clavicular) portion of the pectoralis major share the actions of shoulder flexion, internal rotation, and horizontal adduction. Lying deep to these muscles, the coracobrachialis can assist with shoulder flexion and horizontal adduction. The lower (sternal) portion of the pectoralis major can produce internal rotation and horizontal adduction, as well as shoulder extension when

Table 3.3 Major Upper-Extremity Joint Movements and Muscles

Joint movement	Primary muscles	Secondary muscles
Shoulder flexion	Anterior deltoid Pectoralis major (clavicular)	Coracobrachialis Biceps brachii
Shoulder extension	Latissimus dorsi Teres major Pectoralis major (sternal)	Posterior deltoid Triceps brachii (long head)
Shoulder abduction	Middle deltoid Supraspinatus	Anterior deltoid Pectoralis major (clavicular, upper ranges) Biceps brachii (when shoulder is externally rotated)
Shoulder adduction	Pectoralis major with latissimus dorsi	Posterior deltoid Anterior deltoid Teres major Coracobrachialis Biceps brachii (short head) Triceps brachii (long head)
Shoulder external rotation	Infraspinatus Teres minor	Posterior deltoid
Shoulder internal rotation	Subscapularis Teres major	Anterior deltoid Pectoralis major Latissimus dorsi
Shoulder horizontal abduction	Infraspinatus Teres minor Posterior deltoid	Middle deltoid (posterior fibers) Teres major Latissimus dorsi
Shoulder horizontal adduction	Pectoralis major Anterior deltoid Coracobrachialis	Biceps brachii (short head) (when elbow is extended)
Scapular elevation	Upper trapezius Levator scapulae Rhomboids	N/A
Scapular depression	Lower trapezius Serratus anterior (lower fibers)	Pectoralis minor
Scapular abduction (protraction)	Serratus anterior	Pectoralis minor
Scapular adduction (retraction)	Trapezius Rhomboids	Levator scapulae
Scapular upward rotation	Serratus anterior Trapezius	N/A
Scapular downward rotation	Rhomboids	Levator scapulae Pectoralis minor
Elbow flexion	Biceps brachii Brachialis	Brachioradialis Pronator teres
Elbow extension	Triceps brachii	Anconeus

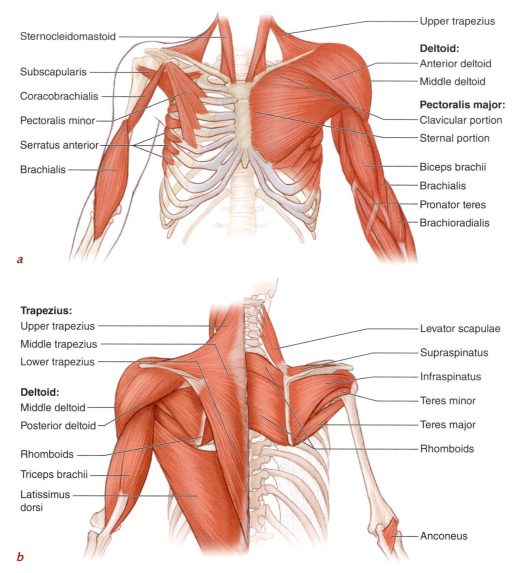

Figure 3.4   Major muscles of the upper extremities: *(a)* front view; *(b)* back view. Deeper muscles are shown on the right side of the body.

the arm is raised to the front. Moving toward the outside, the middle deltoid has a primary action of shoulder abduction. The anterior deltoid can also assist with shoulder abduction.

Looking at a back view of the muscles, the posterior deltoid, latissimus dorsi, and teres major all have actions of shoulder extension and can produce shoulder horizontal abduction. However, they differ in that the posterior deltoid has an action of shoulder external rotation, while the other two muscles traverse to attach to the front of the humerus and so have an action of shoulder internal rotation.

Unlike the hip joint, the shoulder does not have a group of muscles on the inside that are designed for adduction. Instead, a muscle from the front of the shoulder must be paired with a muscle from the back of the shoulder so that their cocontraction results in adduction. The pectoralis major and latissimus dorsi are a strong pair of muscles and are commonly used, but many other pairs can also assist with this movement.

In addition to these muscles, the rotator cuff and scapular muscles aid with movements of the shoulder, often in a less obvious manner. The rotator cuff consists of four small muscles that span between the scapula and upper humerus. The primary function of these muscles is to maintain stability of the shoulder joint. Furthermore, one muscle, the supraspinatus, is a prime mover for shoulder abduction, while the others can produce shoulder external rotation (the teres minor and infraspinatus) or internal rotation (the subscapularis). The teres minor and infraspinatus can also produce the specialized movement of horizontal abduction. Adequate strength of the rotator cuff is vital for correct mechanics of the shoulder and injury prevention. Although isolated strengthening of these muscles is not emphasized in the classical Pilates mat work, exercises for strengthening these muscles are found in mat work, with elastic bands adding resistance. Furthermore, many of the advanced mat exercises requiring that the body weight be supported by the arms, such as Twist (page 164), can have some strength and stability benefits for the rotator cuff in a more functional manner.

The scapular muscles produce movements of the scapula, not the humerus. However, these movements of the scapula are naturally linked with movements of the shoulder and function to promote optimal mechanics of the shoulder. Movements of the scapula are described in chapter 2 (figure 2.11, page 24). A few general principles to keep in mind are that the scapular muscles located on the back of the body, especially the trapezius and rhomboids, act to pull the scapula toward the spine and so produce scapular adduction, while those on the front, the serratus anterior and pectoralis minor, produce the opposite movement of scapular abduction. Those muscles whose fibers run upward from the scapula to attach onto the neck or upper back—the levator scapulae, upper trapezius, and rhomboids—tend to pull the scapula upward to produce scapular elevation, while the lower trapezius, lower fibers of the serratus anterior, and pectoralis minor tend to produce scapular depression. The line of pull relative to their attachment onto the scapula determines what type of rotation they tend to produce, with the serratus anterior and trapezius producing upward rotation, and the others, particularly the rhomboids, producing downward rotation.

The elbow is a hinge joint with the movements of flexion and extension. The two-bellied biceps brachii and the brachialis (located deep relative to the biceps brachii, with its muscle belly extending lower) are on the front of the arm and are the primary flexors of the elbow. Two other muscles that cross the front of the elbow and primarily act to produce movements of the forearm, the brachioradialis and pronator teres, can also assist with elbow flexion. The triceps brachii is on the back of the upper arm and is the most powerful elbow extensor. A small muscle that crosses the back of the elbow, the anconeus, can assist with elbow extension. Portions of the biceps brachii and triceps brachii also cross the shoulder joint and can assist with various movements of the shoulder.

Muscles at Work in Full-Body Movements

When functional movements such as walking, running, or more complex mat exercises are performed, a single muscle does not work in isolation. Instead, such movements involve a symphony of muscles acting in a highly coordinated manner to affect the desired movement. Understanding the types of muscle contractions that can occur, the varying roles muscles can play, and the ability of muscles to work together in a force couple (see page 41) will allow a better appreciation of full-body movements.

Types of Muscle Contraction

Although a standard method to learn the actions of muscles is to deduce the actions they produce when they shorten, not all muscle contractions actually result in visible shortening of a muscle. Although the muscle cells are actively producing tension, depending on the ratio of the forces related to the contracting muscle and the opposing resistance, the muscle as a whole may shorten, lengthen, or stay the same. Muscle contractions can be categorized as dynamic or static.

Dynamic Muscle Contraction

A *dynamic* (historically termed *isotonic*) muscle contraction or tension occurs when the involved muscle changes in length and visible joint movement occurs. A dynamic muscle contraction can be either concentric or eccentric. A concentric muscle contraction involves a shortening of the muscle, with joint movement in the direction of the action of the primary muscle. When gravity provides the resistance, a concentric contraction occurs when the joint moves in the direction opposite to the effect of gravity, often the up phase of the movement. For example, when you perform Chest Lift (page 54), the abdominals act with a concentric contraction to produce the spinal flexion that lifts the upper torso off the mat in the up phase of the movement.

In contrast, an eccentric muscle contraction involves a lengthening of the muscle (i.e., the distance between the attachments of the muscle to the bones becomes greater), with movement in the direction opposite to that of the action of the primary muscle. When gravity provides the resistance, an eccentric contraction occurs when the joint moves in the direction of gravity, often the down phase of the movement. For example, when you perform Chest Lift, the abdominals (spinal flexors) act with an eccentric contraction to control the lowering of the trunk on the down phase of the movement.

This is an important concept to understand, both to analyze movement and perform Pilates mat work with optimal technique. One might think that the spinal extensors are used to produce spinal extension on the down phase of Chest Lift. However, if the extensors were used, your head and torso would crash into the mat. Instead, the same muscles that work on the up phase, the spinal flexors or abdominals, are used eccentrically to smoothly lower the trunk back to the mat with control. Eccentric contractions also commonly occur in faster movements to decelerate a body segment before reversing the direction of movement.

Static Muscle Contraction

With a *static,* or *isometric,* muscle contraction, there is no visible change in muscle length or observable joint movement. Although the muscle is generating tension, the effect of the muscle contraction is exactly counterbalanced by the effect of the resistance, resulting in no net movement. Static muscle contractions are used frequently in Pilates to prevent undesired movement of body segments or to help achieve a desired line of the limbs or other body segments. For example, when you perform Push-Up (page 145), static contractions of muscles at the knees, hips, and spine are essential for keeping the sides of the shoulders, pelvis, and knees in the desired straight-line relationship.

Muscle Roles

Muscles can function in many potential roles. A given muscle does not have a set role but instead can act in different roles with different movements.

The *mover,* or *agonist,* is a muscle that produces the desired movement at a given joint. Movers can be subdivided further into primary and secondary movers or muscles. As previously described, a primary mover is a muscle that is particularly important for producing the desired movement, whereas a secondary mover is a muscle that is less effective but can assist in producing the desired movement.

An *antagonist* is a muscle whose action is directly opposite to the desired movement of the agonist. In many movements, the antagonist does not work, but rather relaxes. In some types of movement, lack of firing of the antagonist is a sign of a higher skill level that allows for more efficient movement. Some Pilates mat exercises fall into this category, in which the goal is to fire the agonist at the optimal time and with just the right amount of force so that the antagonist is not required to stop or help control the movement. However, when a body part must be held rigid (during deceleration of a body part or when extreme precision is required), antagonists often work together with agonists. This coordinated synchronous use is termed *cocontraction*. Cocontraction is also commonly used in Pilates mat work, such as when the abdominals and spinal extensors cocontract, as described in chapter 2.

The term *synergist* can refer to a muscle that acts at the same time as a prime mover to neutralize an undesired secondary action of that mover. An example is given in chapter 2; the lower trapezius acts as a synergist, with its action of depression serving to neutralize the undesired elevation of the upper trapezius while leaving its desired action of upward rotation of the scapula (figure 2.12, page 24).

A *stabilizer* is a muscle that contracts isometrically to support or steady a body part against forces related to a given movement. The contraction of the abdominals to help maintain core stability is discussed in chapter 2 and is a vital part of Pilates mat work.

Muscles Acting as Force Couples

Force couples are muscles located in different positions relative to the axis of a joint but that act together to produce rotation or joint movement in the same direction. One that is particularly important in Pilates mat work is the abdominal–hamstring force couple (figure 3.5). Because of the lower attachment of the abdominals onto the pelvis, contraction of the abdominals can produce a posterior pelvic tilt. Similarly, the attachments of the hamstrings onto the bottom of the back of the pelvis allow them to create a posterior pelvic tilt. So even though these muscles are located on opposite sides of the pelvis, together they act to create the same movement: a posterior rotation of the pelvis. Sometimes in mat work, such as Pelvic Curl (page 52), this action is used to create a posterior pelvic tilt. But in many other exercises this force couple is used to prevent an undesired anterior pelvic tilt (figure 3.5*a*) and maintain a neutral pelvis (figure 3.5*b*). Different cues can encourage use of this force couple, such as "Focus on pulling the lower attachment of the abdominals upward as the hamstrings pull downward."

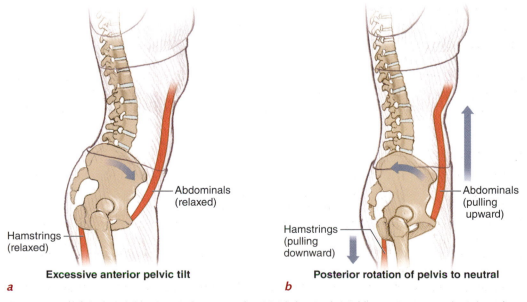

Abdominals (relaxed)

Hamstrings (relaxed)

Excessive anterior pelvic tilt

a

Abdominals (pulling upward)

Hamstrings (pulling downward)

Posterior rotation of pelvis to neutral

b

Figure 3.5 Abdominal–hamstring force couple. *(a)* Abdominals and hamstrings are relaxed, and the force couple is inoperative. *(b)* The force couple acts to rotate the pelvis posteriorly to the desired neutral position.

Movement Analysis of Mat Work

Now it is time to apply the information in this chapter to analyzing mat exercises. A common approach is to examine the movement, focus on the primary joint or joints undergoing movement, and theorize which muscle groups should be active in order to produce or control the movement. With Pilates mat work, gravity provides the primary external resistance. To theorize the muscles that are acting, one must look at the joint movement occurring in various phases of the exercise and the relationship of this movement to gravity during these phases. If the movement goes against gravity, the muscle group that has the same action as the movement will be working concentrically. If the movement goes in the same direction as gravity, the muscle group that has the opposite action as the movement will be working eccentrically.

Let's use Back Extension Prone (page 66) as an example. Visual examination of the movement reveals that the spine is the primary site of action and that spinal extension occurs on the up phase. Since this is the phase that is working against gravity, we know that the muscles whose action is the same as the direction of movement will be working—that is, the spinal extensors are working concentrically. Visual examination of the down phase reveals spinal flexion. However, since in this phase the body is moving in the same direction as gravity, we know that the muscles whose action is opposite to the direction of the movement will be working to control the movement—that is, the spinal extensors are working eccentrically. Examples of the spinal extensors include the erector spinae, semispinalis, and deep posterior spinal group. So, in a simple up and down movement like this, the same muscle group will be working concentrically on the up phase and eccentrically on the down phase. A summary chart for this movement analysis is shown in figure 3.6.

More comprehensive movement analyses may include information on key muscles acting in roles other than movers, such as stabilizers or synergists. When antagonists play an important role in joint stabilization, deceleration, or precision, they also may be included. In some exercises that involve a large range of motion, antagonists may be mentioned if they undergo a dynamic stretch, useful for improving flexibility. Alternatively, the antagonists may provide constraints at the end range of the movement that limit the desired form, particularly in people with tight muscles.

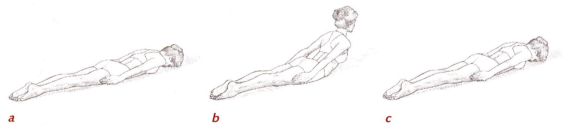

Movement phase	Joint movement	Contraction type	Movers: muscle group (sample muscles)
Up phase, a to b	Spinal extension	Concentric	Spinal extensors (erector spinae, semispinalis, deep posterior spinal group)
Down phase, b to c	Spinal flexion	Eccentric	Spinal extensors (erector spinae, semispinalis, deep posterior spinal group)

Figure 3.6 Anatomical analysis of Back Extension Prone.

The following principles may aid in analyzing a mat exercise. The first principles focus on determining the movers that are responsible for the given movement. The last two principles provide examples of how inadequate strength or flexibility of key muscles can prevent proper execution of a mat exercise and what modifications can help remedy the situation.

- **Muscle group versus specific muscles.** In the initial steps of the movement analysis, determine the muscle group that is working at the joint under consideration (e.g., spinal flexors or hip flexors). Then view examples of specific muscles in that group as seen in tables 3.1 to 3.3. This will allow you to readily check your logic, and it is a simple way to determine muscle use.

- **Movement terminology in different positions.** Although movement terminology is generated from anatomical position, the same terms are used when the body changes its position in space. It is important to think of the movement relative to the body rather than relative to the space you are in. So, raising the arm in a forward direction relative to the body (chest) is termed shoulder flexion whether you are standing, sitting, or lying on your back.

- **Direction of movement versus position.** When visually analyzing a movement, focus on the direction of movement of a given joint rather than the joint position. For example, when bringing the arms from overhead up toward the ceiling in the second phase of Roll-Up (page 73), the upper arms are moving in a backward direction relative to the chest, and so the movement is shoulder extension, even though if you were to stop the movement, the arms would be in a position of shoulder flexion.

- **Open and closed kinematic chain.** In the human body, a kinematic, or kinetic, chain refers to a series of joints that link successive body segments. With many movements of the limbs, the end segment (the hand or foot) moves freely in space, such as when raising the arm to the front. This is termed an open kinematic chain movement. In contrast, in some movements the end segment is fixed, such as when performing a push-up. This is termed a closed kinematic chain. Although the movements look quite different, for movement analysis purposes it is important to focus on the direction of movement of the limb (the upper arm in this case) relative to the trunk when going against gravity. In both instances the shoulder flexors are the prime movers. Closed kinematic chain exercises have been integrated into many training approaches because they require the coordination of multiple joints and often replicate patterns that are valuable for improving activities of daily living.

- **Changing effects of gravity.** Some mat exercises are complex, and changes in the relationship to gravity necessitate changes in the muscles functioning and the type of contraction necessary to produce or control the movement. For example, during Rollover With Legs Spread (page 112), the hip flexors work concentrically to raise the legs (figure 3.7a on page 44). However, as the legs pass vertical, gravity will tend to create hip flexion rather than extension, so the hip extensors must be used to keep the legs from dropping toward the mat. If the angle of the hip remains the same, an isometric contraction of the hip extensors would be utilized (figure 3.7b). Then, when the legs reach their full overhead position, the hip extensors are used eccentrically to control the lowering of the legs toward the mat (figure 3.7c). Lastly, toward the end of the exercise after the pelvis has returned to the mat and the legs have crossed vertical again, gravity tends to create hip extension once more. Now the hip flexors work eccentrically to help control the lowering of the legs (figure 3.7d). So from a movement analysis perspective, to understand which muscles are operative, it is essential to note the relationship of key body segments to gravity in different phases of the movement.

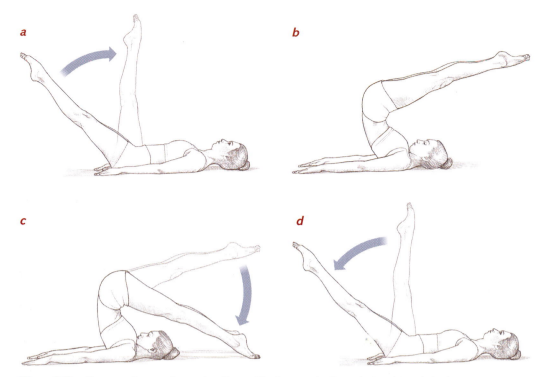

Figure 3.7   Changes in muscle contraction with changes in the relationship of the legs to gravity. *(a)* Concentric use of hip flexors to lift legs to vertical. *(b)* Isometric use of hip extensors to maintain angle at hip joint as spine flexes and shoulders extend. *(c)* Eccentric use of hip extensors to control lowering legs toward the mat. *(d)* Eccentric use of hip flexors to control lowering legs from vertical to start position.

• **Torque.** For most synovial joints, when a muscle contracts it produces rotation of a body segment about the axis going through a joint, resulting in flexion, abduction, external rotation, dorsiflexion, or other joint movements. This is termed *rotary motion,* and the effectiveness of a force to produce rotation is termed *torque.* Torque can be defined as the amount of force multiplied by the moment of force, defined as the perpendicular distance from the line of force to the axis of rotation. In Pilates mat work, this principle is very important for both exercise effectiveness and safety. In essence, the weight of the limbs is the same, but moving them closer or farther away from the trunk markedly affects the torque they exert and the amount of muscle force that must be generated. Hence, performing Chest Lift (page 54) with the hands laced behind the head is much more challenging for the abdominals than performing the same exercise with the arms reaching forward alongside the legs.

The issue of torque is even more important with the legs, because the weight of the legs is so much greater than the arms. So, when you perform Hundred (page 78), the farther the legs move away from vertical (figure 3.8), the greater their moment of force and the greater the torque they will generate. This requires the hip flexors to work harder to counterbalance this greater torque. The required increase in the force of muscle contraction can be quite large because a muscle's line of force tends to run quite close to joints, resulting in a small moment of force. If the abdominals are not working adequately, this forceful contraction of the hip flexors, particularly the iliopsoas, can anteriorly tilt the

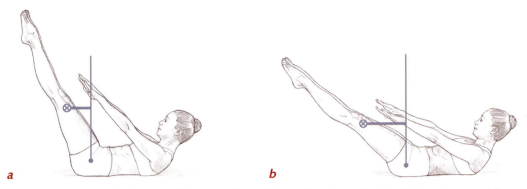

Figure 3.8 Increase in torque with change from *(a)* legs close to vertical to *(b)* legs lower and farther away from vertical.

pelvis and pull the lumbar spine into hyperextension, a potentially injurious situation for the lower back. When performing any exercise in which the legs are held off the mat, it is essential that you select a leg height at which you can consistently maintain stability of the pelvis and lumbar spine to both protect your body from injury and get the most benefit from the exercise.

- **Multijoint muscles and flexibility.** Muscles such as the hamstrings can easily reach their limit of extensibility when they are stretched across two or more joints. For the hamstrings, it is the combination of hip flexion and knee extension that requires the muscles to elongate, and many exercises in mat work incorporate this combination with sitting (Spine Stretch, page 98), bringing the legs overhead (Rollover With Legs Spread, page 112), or holding a V position with the legs off the mat (Rocker With Open Legs, page 108). People with inadequate hamstring flexibility initially must use modifications, such as slightly bending the knees or using a lower hand position for Rocker With Open Legs so that body alignment is not excessively disrupted and the intended benefits of the exercise can be gained.

Understanding Mat Exercise Descriptions

Specific Pilates mat exercises are described in chapters 4 through 9 using the following format.

- **Exercise name.** Whenever possible, the name of the exercise is the name originally used by Joseph Pilates as indicated in *Return to Life Through Contrology*. In some cases, we provide an alternative in parentheses that reflects a name more commonly used by one or more schools of training. Some exercises included in this book are not described in *Return to Life Through Contrology*. These exercise are indicated in the exercise finder at the end of the book.

- **Exercise level.** Exercises are listed as fundamental, intermediate, or advanced based on complexity and difficulty. However, individual differences greatly influence the difficulty of an exercise. Therefore, it is important to judge the level for your own body, based on your experience of doing the exercise and your physical limitations.

- **Execution.** The basic steps for executing the exercise are provided, with their associated breath pattern. Simplified terminology for positions and movements of the body is purposely used in these descriptions to help readers with less anatomical background understand the desired movement sequence. These steps are accompanied by illustrations for added clarity.

In general, the positions shown in the illustrations and described in the steps are similar to those used in *Return to Life Through Contrology*. In some cases, a change was made to be more consistent with current scientific understanding of exercise safety and body alignment. For example, various exercises described in *Return to Life Through Contrology*, such as Hundred (page 78), begin by lifting the legs straight up from the mat. In this book, a starting position with the legs 60 degrees off the mat is commonly used to reduce the torque produced by the legs and help reduce the potential stress on the lower back.

- **Targeted and accompanying muscles.** The targeted and accompanying muscles required for executing the given exercise are listed. As is customary with movement analysis, the list of muscles refers to movement from the starting position and generally does not address the muscles needed to sustain the starting position. This list focuses on movers but often includes key stabilizers and, on occasion, synergists.

For purposes of simplicity, this book focuses only on the key muscles of the spine, hip, knee, ankle, shoulder, and elbow. In terms of the shoulder, generally just the basic movements of shoulder flexion, extension, abduction, and adduction are included, although many mat exercises include subtle shifts of external and internal rotation as the arm moves in space. Similarly, whenever the arm moves, the movement at the shoulder joint is naturally accompanied by linked movements of the scapula that are vital for maintaining optimal technique and proper positioning of the head of the humerus in the socket. Generally, reference to these scapular motions is not included except when they are key for preventing alignment problems commonly associated with a particular exercise.

Because Joseph Pilates did not emphasize the pelvic floor muscles in his original work, reference to these muscles is included only in Pelvic Curl (page 52). It is left to the discretion of the reader to add focused use of the pelvic floor muscles to additional exercises. Furthermore, it is assumed that the deep muscles of core stabilization, including the transversus abdominis and multifidi, are working in the mat exercises, even when not explicitly stated.

As mentioned, the key muscles are broken into two categories—targeted and accompanying muscles. In the main anatomical illustrations, the targeted muscles are illustrated in a darker red, and the accompanying muscles are in a lighter red.

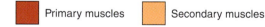

The targeted muscle groups are listed first to help the reader focus on these particularly important muscles. For these targeted muscle groups (e.g., hip flexors and spinal extensors), in general both primary and secondary muscles are listed, while only primary muscles are listed for the accompanying muscle groups. Similarly, within a targeted muscle group, the components of a primary muscle that has multiple parts are listed in parentheses, but the components of the secondary muscles of the targeted group are not listed. For example, if the spinal extensors are targeted, the components of the erector spinae (spinalis, longissimus, and iliocostalis) are listed in parentheses, but the components of the semispinalis and deep posterior spinal group are not. This approach provides greater detail for the most essential muscles in a given exercise while avoiding making the list of key muscles too long or cumbersome.

These key muscles generally correspond to the primary and secondary movers listed in tables 3.1, 3.2, and 3.3. However, in select cases a Pilates exercise may involve a position that reduces the effectiveness of a muscle that is generally considered a primary muscle, and a muscle that is generally considered secondary may take on a primary role. In such cases, the list of muscles under a given Pilates exercise may differ slightly from that provided in the tables.

Furthermore, selection of the most important muscles in Pilates mat exercises is much more subjective and complex than in other training systems such as weight training. With weight training, the muscle group producing the movement required to lift the heavy weight is the targeted muscle group that will be strengthened. In contrast, since Pilates mat work does not incorporate outside resistance other than gravity, its effectiveness for strengthening many muscles is debatable as well as dependent on the participant's current fitness level. Instead, as described in chapter 2, many of the exercises emphasize detailed movement and stabilization of the core, with movement of the limbs functioning more to add a stability challenge than limb strength. Despite these difficulties, an effort has been made to denote muscles that are particularly challenged by a given exercise, using the criteria of muscular strength or muscular endurance when possible. Not surprisingly, the spinal flexors (abdominals) are listed very frequently.

In some exercises that involve a large range of motion, muscles such as the hamstrings or a muscle group such as the hip flexors may undergo a dynamic stretch, potentially useful for improving flexibility. This potential benefit is generally mentioned under exercise notes.

- **Technique cues.** Directives are given to help the reader execute the exercise with optimal technique. More anatomically accurate terminology is used in this section to clarify the key joints that are moving and the related muscles responsible for these movements. The intent of including specific information about the working muscle groups is to foster the development of greater awareness and control of these muscles as they relate to the challenges of the given exercise. Input about the dynamic of the movement is also commonly included. This section often ends with an image, a cue to foster the feeling of the movement that is generally less literal or scientific in nature. Information provided in the technique cues can help you apply the foundation principles of Pilates discussed in chapter 1 and the body alignment principles discussed in chapter 2.

- **Exercise notes.** This category generally includes potential benefits of an exercise as well as discussion about important movement concepts. In many cases this section also includes information on how a particular exercise relates to other exercises that have similar goals or share similar challenges. Cautions may be included for higher-risk exercises.

- **Modifications.** For some exercises in which strength, flexibility, or coordination are common limiting factors, one or more modifications are provided to help address these limitations. For example, if strength is a concern, a modification may be provided to bring the legs closer to vertical or bring the arms in closer to the trunk so that the limbs produce less torque. If hamstring flexibility is a concern, allowing the knees to bend may be a possible modification. If coordination is an issue, focusing on gaining proficiency in easier exercises that focus on the same skill may be recommended. In other cases, breaking the exercise into components and gaining proficiency in the individual elements could be suggested. Using a modification can be a very powerful tool for achieving successful application of the foundation principles of Pilates and preventing injury.

- **Variations.** In an effort to honor the original work of Joseph Pilates, in general the exercises after chapter 4 are presented as they are shown in *Return to Life Through Contrology*. However, today many other variations are common, and selected variations may be described in this section. The variation may include a different breath pattern, body positioning, dynamic, or number of repetitions than that used in the primary exercise description.

Body Aware and Safety Wise

As discussed in chapter 1, the emphasis in Pilates is on the process of how the exercise is performed, not just rushing to execute the most advanced movements. Revel in the sequential mastery of movement skills and the development of body awareness. Don't sacrifice form or have your training come to a screeching halt because of injury.

In some cases, performing a Pilates exercise with optimal technique or waiting until strength, flexibility, and coordination have improved still will not make the exercise appropriate for your body. To provide a historical perspective and a more true representation of the original system, all the mat exercises described in *Return to Life Through Contrology* are included in this book. However, many movement specialists and medical professionals consider some of these exercises inappropriate or at least high risk for the general population. Of particular concern are those exercises that involve lifting both legs off the mat, such as Teaser (page 92); extreme spinal hyperextension, such as Rocking (page 187) and Swan Dive (page 190); and body weight being borne by the neck, such as Control Balance (page 120) and Jackknife (page 123). In the case of the latter, there is risk that a person with low bone density might fracture a vertebra. Although commonly more of concern with older women, for some women the first sign of low bone density is a potentially devastating vertebral fracture. Furthermore, factors such as genetics, exercise history, eating disorders, or other medical conditions can place young, seemingly healthy people at risk.

So before beginning this program, check with your physician to see if you need to avoid certain positions, particularly the ones just listed. Also, listen to your body. If you feel joint discomfort, don't continue the exercise. If the discomfort is mild, check your form and make any needed corrections, perform the exercise with a smaller range of motion, or utilize other appropriate modifications. If the discomfort is more severe or persists after you try modifications, stop performing the exercise immediately, and get medical advice regarding whether it is appropriate for you and, if so, what type of modification would be best for you to use when attempting the exercise again. It is not necessary to be able to perform all the Pilates mat exercises to get profound benefits. If you are not sure something is right for you, it's better to be safe than sorry. Savor the exercises you can do, and don't worry about those that are not right for you at this time. You may be surprised that after your fitness and proficiency improve, exercises that originally were associated with mild discomfort may no longer produce discomfort and may become some of your favorite exercises.

Get ready. In preparation to begin, get any needed medical clearance to help you select appropriate exercises for your body. Review the recommended approach for learning the mat exercises given at the end of chapter 1. Perform a 5- to 10-minute general warm-up that incorporates repetitive use of large muscle groups, such as brisk walking, so that your heart rate and internal temperature are adequately elevated.

Get set. Position yourself on your mat as needed for a given exercise, and think of setting your core stability before any movement of the spine or limbs. For many exercises, this means drawing the abdominal wall inward to encourage activation of the transversus abdominis. For other exercises, it involves a cocontraction of the abdominals and spinal extensors so that the lower back and pelvis stay neutral or move with the desired alignment. Whatever core strategy is needed, the goal is to have a sense of a strong center, no matter the direction of movement.

Go. Perform the movement described in the exercise steps while maintaining a sense of center. Readers with limited Pilates experience should begin with the fundamental movements in chapter 4 and gradually add fundamental exercises from subsequent chapters.

When you have learned the basic patterns, focus on applying the foundation principles discussed in chapter 1 with greater depth and clarity. Refer to chapter 1 repeatedly for help with lateral breathing or a description of the foundation principles. Also, gradually add more precise use of core stability and other alignment principles discussed in chapter 2. As your movement becomes more centered and exhibits more precise control and flow, add more challenging exercises. Finally, proceed to chapter 10 to learn how to build a comprehensive mat work session and to see sample programs that you can adapt to your individual needs and ability.

FOUNDATION FOR
A MAT SESSION

This chapter focuses on exercises that can be performed at the beginning of the mat session. These exercises emphasize the *powerhouse,* discussed in chapter 2, and serve as a specific warm-up to help prepare you for the more challenging Pilates exercises that follow. They also provide an opportunity to shift your mental focus inward, let go of the stressors of everyday life, and develop an inner calmness.

Although they seem simple, do not miss the value of these foundation exercises. In accordance with the physiological principles of a warm-up, these exercises are less complex and less challenging in terms of balance than many exercises from the classic mat work that appear later. Also, these foundation exercises can be performed more slowly and the difficulty adjusted easily by beginning with a smaller range of motion and progressing to a larger range. Hence, these exercises provide a perfect opportunity to focus on more internal and detailed elements of exercise execution—elements that distinguish Pilates from many other exercise systems.

Technique elements covered in this chapter are activation of the pelvic floor muscles, activation of the transversus abdominis muscle, cocontraction of the abdominals and hamstrings to position the pelvis, smooth articulation of the spine to create a C curve, activation of the oblique muscles, and cocontraction of the abdominals when extending (arching) the back. The goal is to learn and rehearse these motor skills so that they can easily be applied to related exercises. Remember that in Pilates the emphasis is on *how* you perform the movements. Quality and precision of execution are important. Simply following the exercise steps is not enough. Application of the technique cues and principles discussed under exercise notes is essential for gaining the full benefit of each exercise.

Although the exercises in this chapter do not appear in *Return to Life Through Contrology* and are not regarded as part of the classic repertoire, they have become standards in many schools of Pilates and are frequently used in mat classes. Despite all being fundamental, the exercises in this chapter are ordered in terms of increasing difficulty. Therefore, the exercises begin with abdominal strengthening and trunk stabilization in which spinal flexion occurs in a stable supine position, followed by lateral flexion in a less stable side-lying position. Spinal rotation is then added. Lastly, when the trunk muscles are adequately prepared, spinal extension is performed.

Because of their placement at the beginning of the workout, each of these exercises should be executed with low to moderate intensity so that the focus is on warming up and finding inner technique connections rather than on maximizing strength gains. Although this order is recommended while learning the skills demanded by these exercises, once adequate proficiency has been achieved, the sequencing and position of some of these exercises in a workout can be changed to meet individual profiles.

Pelvic Curl

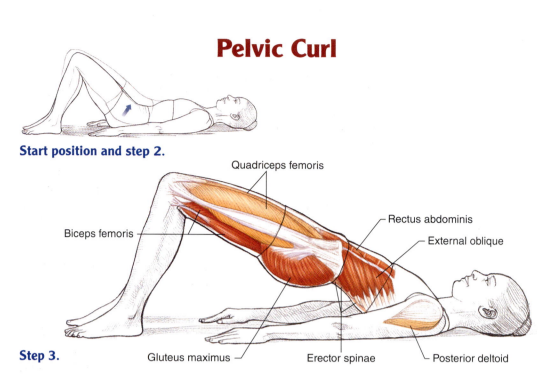

Start position and step 2.

Quadriceps femoris

Rectus abdominis

Biceps femoris

External oblique

Step 3.

Gluteus maximus — Erector spinae — Posterior deltoid

Execution

1. *Start position.* Lie supine with the knees bent and the feet flat on the mat and hip-width apart. Place the arms by the sides with the palms facing down. Focus inward, and consciously relax the neck, shoulders, and lower back muscles while maintaining a neutral pelvic position.

2. *Exhale.* Draw the abdominal wall inward, and slowly curl the pelvis and lower, middle, and upper back sequentially off the mat.

3. *Inhale.* Lift the upper trunk slightly higher to form a straight line on the side of the body running through the shoulder, pelvis, and knee as shown in the main muscle illustration.

4. *Exhale.* Slowly lower the trunk, articulating each vertebra, to return to the start position. Repeat the sequence 10 times.

Targeted Muscles

Spinal flexors: rectus abdominis, external oblique, internal oblique

Anterior spinal stabilizer: transversus abdominis

Pelvic floor muscles: coccygeus, levator ani (pubococcygeus, puborectalis, iliococcygeus)

Hip extensors: gluteus maximus, hamstrings (semitendinosus, semimembranosus, biceps femoris)

Accompanying Muscles

Spinal extensors: erector spinae

Knee extensors: quadriceps femoris

Shoulder extensors: latissimus dorsi, teres major, posterior deltoid

Technique Cues

- In step 2, at the beginning of the exhale, draw the pelvic floor muscles upward and the abdominal wall in toward the spine. This will encourage use of the transversus abdominis just before using the other abdominal muscles that posteriorly tilt the pelvis and flex the spine sequentially from bottom to top as it is curled off the mat.

- Press the feet into the mat, and think of gently pulling the sit bones toward the knees while lifting the bottom of the pelvis to emphasize using the hip extensors, especially the hamstrings. The knee extensors also help raise the thighs upward from the start position.

- In step 3, press the arms down into the mat so the shoulder extensors aid with lifting the upper trunk. Also, focus on activating the upper spinal extensors to align the upper trunk with the shoulders and knees.

- Throughout the movement, keep the knees facing forward.

- *Imagine.* To help achieve the desired motion of the pelvis and spine in step 2, imagine that the area between the rib cage and pubic bone is a shallow bowl. Scoop the abdominal wall inward to touch the inside of the shallow bowl, and then slowly rock that bowl by lifting the bottom rim toward the rib cage.

Exercise Notes

Pelvic Curl can help you learn to focus on activating the deep pelvic floor and transversus abdominis muscles, to sequentially articulate the pelvis and spine, and to cocontract the muscles of the powerhouse in the desired manner.

Focus on the hamstrings. Appropriate contraction of the hamstring muscles is vital for the desired articulation of the pelvis and spine in this exercise. The three hamstring muscles (see the illustration) run down the back of the thigh from the sit bones to below the knee. In this exercise and other similar supine Pilates exercises in which the feet are on the mat in a closed kinematic chain (see chapter 3), the hamstrings produce hip extension by lifting the pelvis rather

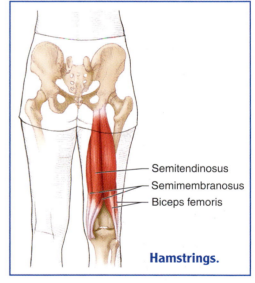

Semitendinosus
Semimembranosus
Biceps femoris

Hamstrings.

than moving the legs. Focusing on lifting the bottom of the pelvis can help utilize these important muscles and prevent the common error of lifting the trunk as a rigid unit or arching the lower back. The coordinated contraction of the hamstrings with the abdominals, termed the abdominal–hamstring force couple (discussed in chapter 3), also serves another important role of helping to rotate the top of the pelvis backward in a posterior pelvic tilt. This function is used in the early part of the exercise to curl the pelvis and later to help maintain a neutral position of the pelvis and assist in countering hyperlordosis.

Chest Lift

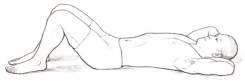

Start position.

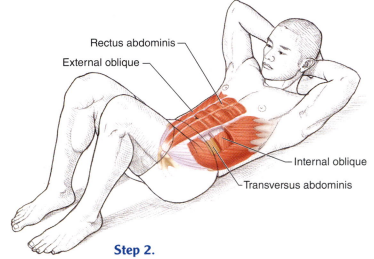

Rectus abdominis

External oblique

Internal oblique

Transversus abdominis

Step 2.

Execution

1. *Start position.* Lie supine with the knees bent and the feet flat on the mat and hip-width apart. Interlace the fingers behind the head, and bend the elbows so they point sideways. Tilt the chin slightly down toward the chest.

2. *Exhale.* Slowly curl the head and upper trunk up, as shown in the main muscle illustration, so that the scapulae lift off the mat while the back portion of the waistline establishes contact with the mat. Pull in the abdominal wall farther, deepening the forward curved position of the trunk.

3. *Inhale.* Pause.

4. *Exhale.* Slowly lower the trunk and head to return to the start position. Repeat the sequence 10 times.

Targeted Muscles

Spinal flexors: rectus abdominis, external oblique, internal oblique

Accompanying Muscles

Anterior spinal stabilizer: transversus abdominis

Technique Cues

- In step 2, at the beginning of the exhale, draw the abdominal wall in toward the spine to encourage use of the transversus abdominis just before using the other abdominals—rectus abdominis, external obliques, and internal obliques—to tilt the pelvis slightly posteriorly, and then flex the spine sequentially from top to bottom.
- Once the head has been lifted in step 2, keep the chin the same distance from the chest and focus on using the abdominals to bring the front of the lower rib cage down toward the front of the pelvis.
- To help target the abdominals, keep the elbows back in line with the shoulders as the trunk is raised into flexion. Avoid swinging the elbows forward, pulling on the head, or using excessive momentum to help raise the trunk.
- During the pause in step 3, focus on lateral breathing (see chapter 1) so that the abdominal wall can remain pulled in and the torso held at the same height despite the inhale.
- In step 4, use the abdominals to control lowering the trunk back to the start position. Focus on pressing one vertebra at a time sequentially into the mat, from the lower to the upper spine, as opposed to lowering rigid sections of the spine.
- *Imagine.* To help achieve the desired flexion of the spine in step 2, imagine the upper and middle trunk curving up and around an exercise ball, with the curve evenly distributed rather than exaggerated in any one region.

Exercise Notes

This relatively simple exercise offers a perfect opportunity to learn how to effectively recruit the abdominals for strength gains and for use in more challenging abdominal exercises.

Create a C curve. The key concept to remember is this: Since the abdominals span between the rib cage and pelvis, effective overload to the abdominals for this exercise entails maximal flexion from the upper back to the beginning of the lower back rather than excessive flexion of the neck or hips. Achieving the desired distributed curvature of the spine, while pulling the abdominal wall in so that it is as concave as possible, can be referred to as creating a C curve of the spine. This terminology will be used to simplify related exercise descriptions.

Variation

As you lift into forward flexion, keep the pelvis in a neutral position instead of creating a slight posterior tilt. This will demand skilled cocontraction of the abdominals and spinal extensors.

Leg Lift Supine

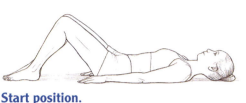

Start position.

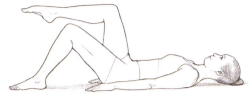

Step 2.

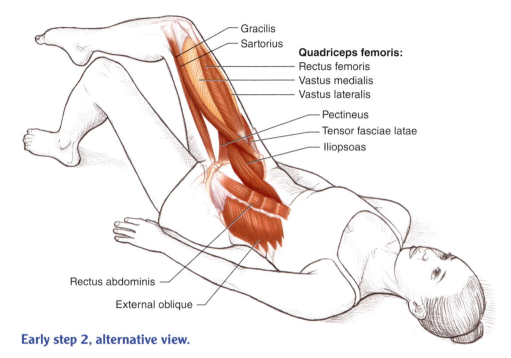

Gracilis
Sartorius

Quadriceps femoris:
Rectus femoris
Vastus medialis
Vastus lateralis

Pectineus
Tensor fasciae latae
Iliopsoas

Rectus abdominis

External oblique

Early step 2, alternative view.

Execution

1. *Start position.* Lie supine with the knees bent so the lower legs form approximately 90-degree angles relative to the thighs and the feet are flat on the mat and hip-width apart. The arms are by the sides with the palms facing down.

2. *Exhale.* Raise one leg until the knee is just above the hip joint, the thigh perpendicular to the mat, while maintaining the 90-degree angle at the knee joint as shown in step 2.

3. *Inhale.* Lower the leg until the toes touch the mat, while still maintaining the 90-degree angle at the knee joint. Repeat the sequence five times with the same leg. Place the foot fully down on the mat. Perform the same sequence with the opposite leg.

Targeted Muscles

Hip flexors: iliopsoas, rectus femoris, sartorius, pectineus, tensor fascia latae, gracilis

Anterior spinal stabilizers: rectus abdominis, external oblique, internal oblique, transversus abdominis

Accompanying Muscles

Knee extensors: quadriceps femoris

Technique Cues

- Focus on keeping the pelvis stationary and the weight evenly distributed on both sides of the pelvis as the hip flexors raise the leg in step 2 and then eccentrically lower the leg in step 3. Avoid shifting weight to the opposite side of the pelvis as the leg lifts and lowers.
- As the leg lifts in step 2, contract the knee extensors to maintain the desired 90-degree angle of the knee and prevent the lower leg from dropping down because of gravity.
- Emphasize isolating the movement to the hip joint, with the leg lifting and lowering with no changes in knee angle or in rib cage or pelvic alignment.
- *Imagine.* To help achieve the desired isolated movement, imagine the cover of a heavy textbook easily closing and opening with no effect on the very heavy and stable body of the text. The leg acts like the cover of the book. You should feel a sense of lightness in the moving leg.

Exercise Notes

This simple but valuable exercise focuses on using the necessary muscles, primarily the abdominals, to keep the trunk stable as the lower limbs move.

Trunk stabilization with hip flexion. In this exercise, the abdominals are working as stabilizers rather than movers. Because the upper attachments of many of the hip flexors are on the sides of the lower spine and the front of the pelvis, when they forcibly contract to lift the leg, they also tend to arch the lower back and pull the front of the pelvis forward into an anterior pelvic tilt, unless adequate stabilization of the pelvis and spine is provided by the abdominals.

Research suggests that the transversus abdominis (see the illustration) plays a particularly important role in stabilization when the limbs move. The fibers of the transversus abdominis run almost horizontal. Therefore, focusing on pulling the deep abdominal wall inward toward the spine can help activate this muscle to maintain the desired neutral position of the pelvis. Building the skill of using the abdominals and other muscles of the powerhouse to stabilize the trunk is an essential goal of Pilates and vital for proper execution of some of the advanced landmark Pilates exercises, such as Teaser (page 92).

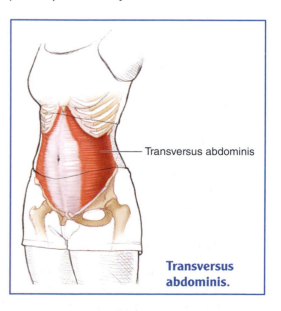

Transversus abdominis

Transversus abdominis.

Leg Lift Side

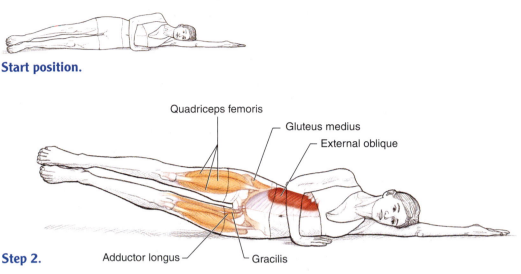

Start position.

Quadriceps femoris

Gluteus medius

External oblique

Step 2.

Adductor longus

Gracilis

Execution

1. *Start position.* Lie on one side, with the bottom arm and both legs straight and in line with the trunk. The head is resting on the bottom arm. The top arm is bent, with the palm on the mat in front of the torso and the fingers pointing toward the head.

2. *Exhale.* Raise both legs as one unit toward the ceiling, and then lift the legs higher by laterally flexing the spine. See the main muscle illustration.

3. *Inhale.* Lower the legs until they are just above, but not touching, the mat. Repeat the sequence 10 times. Lower the legs to the start position. Perform the same sequence on the opposite side.

Targeted Muscles

Lower spinal lateral flexors: external oblique, internal oblique, quadratus lumborum, erector spinae (spinalis, longissimus, iliocostalis), semispinalis, deep posterior spinal group (multifidus, rotatores, intertransversales), iliopsoas

Accompanying Muscles

Hip abductors of top leg: gluteus medius, gluteus minimus

Hip adductors of bottom leg: adductor longus, adductor brevis, adductor magnus, gracilis

Knee extensors: quadriceps femoris

Ankle–foot plantar flexors: gastrocnemius, soleus

Technique Cues

- In step 2, move the legs as one unit by using the hip adductors to pull the bottom leg up against the top leg, while the hip abductors of the top leg raise the top leg. The knee extensors keep both knees straight as the ankle–foot plantar flexors keep both feet pointed.

- Initially focus on the movement occurring at the hip joints while the trunk stays stationary, with the waist lifted off the mat. Then, to lift the legs higher, emphasize activating the lateral flexors of the spine by bringing the side of the pelvis closer to the rib cage on the upper side of the body while the legs reach up toward the ceiling. In this phase, the waist will lower toward the mat as the spine laterally flexes and the pelvis laterally tilts.

- The hips should remain stacked, with the top hip bone vertically above the lower hip bone. Avoid rocking backward or forward as the legs move.

- *Imagine.* To help achieve correct form and movement quality, imagine an archer's bow being pulled tight. As the legs arc up toward the sky, they create a bow shape together with the trunk.

Exercise Notes

Although this exercise can provide some toning benefits for both the hip adductors and abductors, its primary purpose is to strengthen the lateral flexors of the spine and develop essential skills for core stability.

Spinal lateral flexion. Ideally, lateral flexion involves bending the spine directly to the side. This movement requires a finely coordinated simultaneous contraction of muscles located in the front, primarily the obliques and iliopsoas; muscles located on the side, primarily the quadratus lumborum; and muscles located in the back, including the erector spinae, semispinalis, and components of the deep posterior spinal group (see the illustration). With optimal form, the obliques do most of the work, with the back muscles firing just sufficiently to keep the trunk from flexing forward. However, it is common to use too much activation of the back muscles, causing the lower back to arch. In such cases, allow the feet to come forward slightly, and emphasize pulling the abdominal wall inward so the body is in a slight banana shape when viewed from the top to facilitate a more desired use of the obliques.

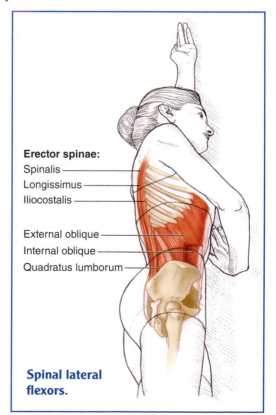

Erector spinae:
Spinalis
Longissimus
Iliocostalis

External oblique
Internal oblique
Quadratus lumborum

Spinal lateral flexors.

Leg Pull Side

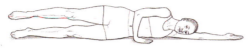

Start position.

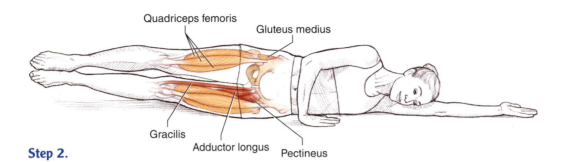

Quadriceps femoris

Gluteus medius

Gracilis

Adductor longus   Pectineus

Step 2.

Execution

1. *Start position.* Lie on one side, with the bottom arm and both legs straight and in line with the trunk. The head is resting on the bottom arm. The top arm is bent, with the palm on the mat in front of the torso, the fingers pointing toward the head. The bottom leg is resting on the mat, and the top leg is held slightly higher than the top hip. Feet are pointed.

2. *Exhale.* Raise the bottom leg toward the top leg, ideally until touching. See the main muscle illustration.

3. *Inhale.* Lower the bottom leg until it lightly touches the mat. Repeat the sequence 10 times. After the last repetition, lower the bottom leg to rest fully on the mat. Perform the same sequence on the other side.

Targeted Muscles

Hip adductors of bottom leg: adductor longus, adductor brevis, adductor magnus, gracilis, pectineus

Accompanying Muscles

Lateral spinal stabilizers and lower spinal lateral flexors: external oblique, internal oblique, quadratus lumborum, erector spinae

Hip abductors of top leg: gluteus medius, gluteus minimus

Knee extensors: quadriceps femoris

Ankle–foot plantar flexors: gastrocnemius, soleus

Technique Cues

- Focus on using the hip abductors to keep the top leg stationary. Use the hip adductors to raise the bottom leg in step 2, and then use them eccentrically to lower the bottom leg in step 3. The knee extensors keep the knees straight while the ankle–foot plantar flexors keep the feet pointed throughout the exercise.

- Keep the waist lifted off the mat and the pelvis still throughout the exercise. By keeping the bottom of the rib cage close to the side of the pelvis with the waist lifted, the spinal lateral flexors of the lower side of the body can be used to limit the lateral tilt of the pelvis. This facilitates greater overload to the hip adductors.

- Keep the hips stacked, and avoid rocking the top hip bone backward or forward.

- *Imagine.* To help achieve the desired isolated movement of the leg at the hip joint, imagine an open protractor facing sideways, with the bottom arm of the protractor rising to close the angle.

Exercise Notes

The purpose of this exercise is to improve muscle strength or tone in the hip adductors while maintaining trunk stability in this challenging side-lying position. If trunk stability cannot be adequately maintained and the back arches or the hips rock back and forth, move the legs slightly forward to create a banana shape, as described in Leg Lift Side (page 58).

The hip adductors (see the illustration) are a massive group of muscles that includes the adductor longus, adductor brevis, adductor magnus, gracilis, and pectineus. All of these, except the pectineus, are considered prime movers for hip adduction. Because of their location, the hip adductors are often referred to as the inner thigh muscles. This popular exercise tones the inner thighs and helps counter the jiggle that can occur during walking when these muscles are out of shape.

The hip adductors are used to raise the bottom leg off the mat in any side-lying exercise, such as Leg Lift Side (page 58). They also are used to keep the legs together in many Pilates exercises in which both legs move in unison, such as Jackknife (page 123) and Corkscrew (page 168). This use of the adductors to keep the legs together as the legs reach out is a key element in achieving the long and connected line of the legs that is vital to the Pilates aesthetic.

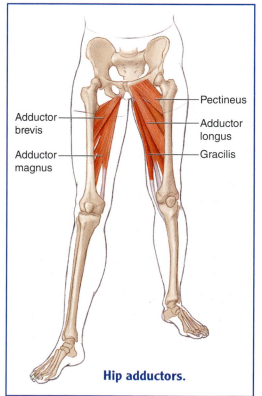

Hip adductors.

Spine Twist Supine

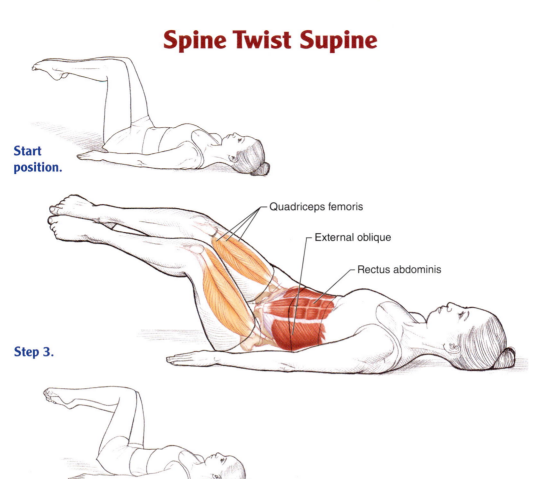

Start position.

Quadriceps femoris

External oblique

Rectus abdominis

Step 3.

Step 5.

Execution

1. *Start position.* Lie supine with the hips and knees at 90-degree angles so that the knees are directly above the hip joints and the lower legs are parallel to the mat. Feet are gently pointed. The arms are straight down by the sides, with the palms facing down.

2. *Exhale.* Pull the abdominal wall in, and perform a slight posterior pelvic tilt. Gently pull the inner thighs together.

3. *Inhale.* Rotate the middle and lower trunk so that the pelvis and knees move as a single unit to one side as shown in the main muscle illustration.

4. *Exhale.* Rotate back to center.

5. *Inhale.* Rotate the middle and lower trunk to the opposite side as shown, moving the pelvis and knees as one unit.

6. *Exhale.* Rotate back to center. Repeat the sequence five times each direction.

Targeted Muscles

Spinal flexors and rotators: rectus abdominis, external oblique, internal oblique, transversus abdominis

Accompanying Muscles

Spinal extensors and rotators: erector spinae

Hip flexors: iliopsoas, rectus femoris

Hip horizontal adductors: adductor longus, adductor brevis, adductor magnus, pectineus

Knee extensors: quadriceps femoris

Ankle–foot plantar flexors: gastrocnemius, soleus

Technique Cues

- In step 2, focus on drawing the transversus abdominis inward and using the obliques to rotate the trunk so the pelvis and knees go to one side while the shoulders remain stationary and in full contact with the mat in step 3.
- Further deepen the flexion of the lower spine before pulling the lower side of the pelvis back toward the opposite side of the rib cage in step 4. This encourages greater use of the obliques, not the spinal extensors, to produce the rotation.
- Pull the knees together gently, using the hip horizontal adductors to keep the bottom leg lifted as the spine rotates. Keep the knees aligned with the center of the pelvis as the ankle–foot plantar flexors keep the feet pointed throughout the exercise.
- Maintain the 90-degree angles at the hips and knees throughout the exercise.
- *Imagine.* To help achieve the desired motion of the pelvis and spine, imagine a steering wheel turning slowly in one direction and then the other.

Exercise Notes

This exercise is valuable for learning to rotate the pelvis and lower back while maintaining desired alignment of the core. When rotating the spine, the common error is to excessively arch the back so the spinal extensors, not the abdominals, primarily affect the movement. Learning to use the transversus abdominis and obliques in this supine position can help protect the spine from injury when spinal rotation is used, particularly in more challenging exercises or during athletic activities.

Tabletop position. The tabletop position shown in step 1 is one of the fundamental supine positions used in Pilates. In this position, the hip flexors help maintain the 90-degree angles at the hips and prevent the legs from moving away from the chest. The knee extensors are used to create the 90-degree angles at the knees and to prevent the lower legs from dropping down to the mat.

Variation

Keep the pelvis in a neutral position as the spine rotates and the pelvis tips onto its side. This will change the desired muscle recruitment to an intricate cocontraction of the abdominals and the spinal extensors.

Chest Lift With Rotation

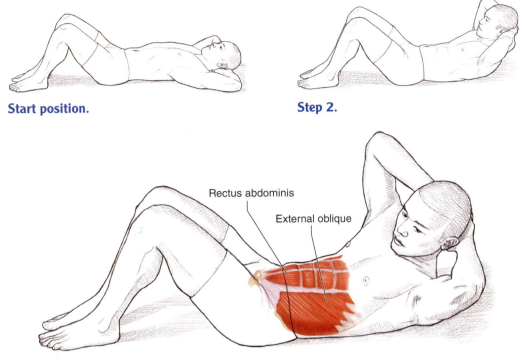

Start position.

Step 2.

Rectus abdominis

External oblique

Step 4.

Execution

1. *Start position.* Start in the same position as for Chest Lift (page 54), supine with the knees bent and feet flat on the mat and hip-width apart. Interlace the fingers behind the head, and bend the elbows so they point to the sides. The chin is tilted slightly down toward the chest.
2. *Exhale.* Slowly curl the head and upper trunk up as shown so that the scapulae lift off the mat while the back of the waistline contacts the mat.
3. *Inhale.* Pause.
4. *Exhale.* Rotate the upper trunk to one side. See the main muscle illustration.
5. *Inhale.* Rotate back to center.
6. *Exhale.* Rotate the upper trunk to the opposite side.
7. *Inhale.* Rotate back to center. Continue alternating the rotation 10 times (5 times each side) while the head and upper trunk remain lifted off the mat. On the last repetition, pause in the center, pulling the abdominal wall farther inward, and then slowly exhale while lowering the trunk and head to the start position.

Targeted Muscles

Spinal flexors and rotators: rectus abdominis, external oblique, internal oblique, transversus abdominis

Technique Cues

- Use the abdominals to maintain a slight posterior tilt of the pelvis, the desired C curve of the spine, and the desired height of the trunk off the mat while the upper trunk rotates from side to side.
- Once the head has been lifted in step 2, maintain the same degree of neck flexion with the elbows in line with the shoulders so that the focus is on using the obliques to rotate the upper trunk while the pelvis remains stationary in steps 4 through 7.
- Avoid bringing the elbows forward and pulling on the head, or bringing the chin farther down or forward.
- At the end of step 7, use the abdominals eccentrically to create a smooth, sequential lowering of the trunk and head back to the start position.
- *Imagine.* To help achieve the desired trunk rotation, imagine the trunk lifting as it rotates, like the swell of a wave. Keep both sides of the trunk long, and avoid bending the trunk to the side.

Exercise Notes

This basic exercise is valuable for developing the obliques, muscles essential for providing contour and tone in the abdominal area to the sides of the central rectus abdominis. The obliques also play a key role in trunk stability and prevention of lower back injury, and are fundamental to most athletic activities.

Oblique focus. Because many muscles can produce rotation, keeping the C curve with the spine flexed rather than flattening during rotation will effectively challenge the obliques. In addition, note that the upper portion of the external oblique runs from the outside of the rib cage diagonally down toward the central tendon, called the *linea alba* (see the illustration). In contrast, the internal oblique runs diagonally up to attach to the central tendon and the undersurface of the rib cage. So, when rotating the upper trunk to the left, focusing on bringing the right side of the rib cage toward the center and then the center toward the opposite hip bone (left ASIS) can help activate the desired right external and left internal oblique muscles. There should be a sensation of both sides of the abdominal area rigorously working as the upper trunk rotates. The transversus abdominis may also assist with rotation.

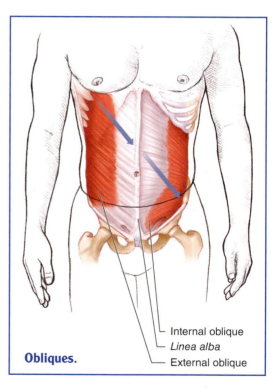

Obliques.

Internal oblique
Linea alba
External oblique

Variation

As the body lifts into forward flexion, keep the pelvis in a neutral position instead of creating a slight posterior tilt.

Back Extension Prone

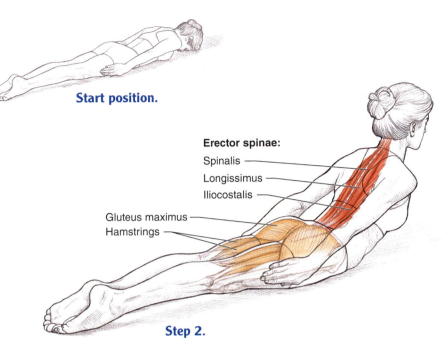

Start position.

Erector spinae:
Spinalis
Longissimus
Iliocostalis
Gluteus maximus
Hamstrings

Step 2.

Execution

1. *Start position.* Lie prone with the forehead on the mat and the arms by the sides with the palms pressing against the sides of the thighs, elbows straight. The legs should be together with the feet gently pointed.
2. *Exhale.* Lift the head, upper trunk, and middle trunk off the mat while keeping the legs together and the arms pressing against the sides. See the main muscle illustration.
3. *Inhale.* Slowly lower the trunk and head, returning to the start position. Repeat the sequence 10 times.

Targeted Muscles

Spinal extensors: erector spinae (spinalis, longissimus, iliocostalis), semispinalis, deep posterior spinal group

Accompanying Muscles

Anterior spinal stabilizers: transversus abdominis, internal oblique, external oblique, rectus abdominis

Hip extensors: gluteus maximus, hamstrings

Shoulder adductors: latissimus dorsi, pectoralis major

Elbow extensors: triceps brachii

Technique Cues

- In step 2, maintain abdominal support, and keep the legs together and in contact with the mat as the spinal extensors are used to raise the upper trunk.

- Focus on sequentially extending the back, vertebra by vertebra, starting from the top, particularly emphasizing the spinal extensors in the upper and middle back while continuing to reach the head out in line with the upper back.

- Continue pressing the arms against the sides using the shoulder adductors, particularly the latissimus dorsi and pectoralis major. Both of these muscles can also help depress the shoulders, so reaching the fingertips gently down toward the feet while the elbow extensors keep the elbows straight can help activate them. Recruitment of the latissimus dorsi is desirable because it is a key muscle for trunk stabilization.

- In step 3, use the spinal extensors eccentrically to control lowering the trunk, this time sequentially from bottom to top, while the abdominals continue to provide support.

- *Imagine.* To achieve the desired feeling of elongation, imagine a rubber band anchored at one end (your feet) being pulled out and up from the other end (the crown of your head).

Exercise Notes

The purpose of this exercise is to strengthen the spinal extensors, particularly the erector spinae, while working on developing the ability to simultaneously use the abdominals to help protect the lower back.

Abdominal support with spinal extension. Because the lower back, or lumbar, curve is concave posteriorly but the upper back, or thoracic, curve is concave anteriorly, the tendency is predominantly to arch the lower back when performing this and similar spinal extension exercises. Arching the lower back also tends to be linked with tilting the top of the pelvis forward to create an anterior pelvic

(continued)

Back Extension Prone   *(continued)*

tilt (see the first illustration below). However, pulling the lower attachment of the abdominals upward can produce rotation of the pelvis in the opposite direction, a posterior pelvic tilt (see the second illustration below). Think of gently pressing the pubic bone into the mat while the lower portion of the abdominals pulls up and in toward the spine to limit the amount of anterior pelvic tilt and reduce the stress to the vulnerable lower lumbar spine. This stabilization of the lower back also facilitates focusing on and strengthening the upper back muscles, which are key for preventing slumped posture. The hip extensors may also help stabilize the pelvis and prevent it from tilting forward excessively (the abdominal–hamstring force couple is discussed in chapter 3). Learning to use the abdominals to help stabilize the lower back in this basic exercise is essential for optimal execution of more challenging exercises involving spinal extension, such as Swimming (page 184) and Double Kick (page 181).

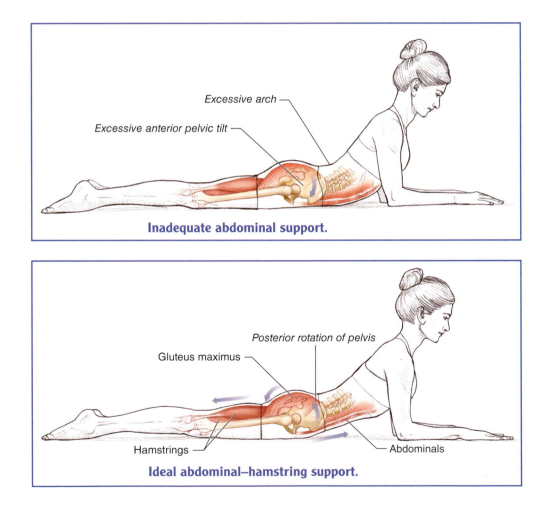

Excessive arch

Excessive anterior pelvic tilt

Inadequate abdominal support.

Posterior rotation of pelvis

Gluteus maximus

Hamstrings

Abdominals

Ideal abdominal–hamstring support.

ABDOMINAL WORK FOR MOVEMENT AND STABILIZATION

As discussed in chapter 2, the abdominals are vital to the Pilates concept of the power-house. They also are a key element in the more current and related concept of core stability, which is popular both in the area of rehabilitation and the arena of athletic performance enhancement. Although most Pilates exercises encourage use of the abdominals, the exercises in this chapter focus particularly on strengthening the abdominals in their action of spinal flexion and also developing the skill of using the abdominals for stabilization. Many exercises in future chapters apply the strength and skill developed here to exercises that involve more challenging actions of the abdominals, detailed articulation of the spine, and more complex movement sequences.

Pay close attention to technique and precision of performance so that both adequate strength and the desired movement patterns are developed. This is very important. Poor execution will fail to produce the desired results and may result in injury. Furthermore, some exercises are not appropriate for everyone. Check with your physician to see what is appropriate for you, and use modifications whenever necessary. If you take care to start at the appropriate level and gradually progress, you will gain strength and skills that will improve the performance of your Pilates workout and contribute to the many activities of daily living and athletic pursuits. It is also important to recognize that the strength and skills gained can help protect the back from injury.

This chapter includes exercises that use the abdominals in a variety of modes. One-Leg Circle (page 70) focuses on using the abdominals to carefully control movements of the pelvis as one leg undergoes movement in multiple directions. In the closely aligned Roll-Up (page 73) and Neck Pull (page 76), the abdominals are used as prime movers in their action of spinal flexion as well as stabilizers while the legs remain straight, resting on the mat. In the next group of related exercises, the abdominals are used in an isometric manner to maintain a position of spinal flexion while the legs are held out straight (Hundred, page 78) or moved (One-Leg Stretch, page 82; Single Straight-Leg Stretch, page 84; Double-Leg Stretch, page 87) in the air and off the mat. Hundred and Double-Leg Stretch provide the additional challenge of holding both legs or moving both legs simultaneously away from the center while maintaining spinal flexion. Crisscross (page 90) advances the challenge of One-Leg Stretch by adding rotation of the torso while maintaining flexion of the spine. Teaser (page 92) represents the most complex exercise. In addition to both legs being held out simultaneously, the abdominals work to raise and lower the upper trunk rather than hold it still in space.

Many of the exercises in this chapter are closely related. It is valuable to note the similarities and differences when developing the required abdominal strength and stabilization skills. Making such connections can help you transfer skills highlighted in this chapter to related exercises in future chapters as well as when compiling a comprehensive Pilates program, which is discussed further in chapter 10.

One-Leg Circle (Leg Circle)

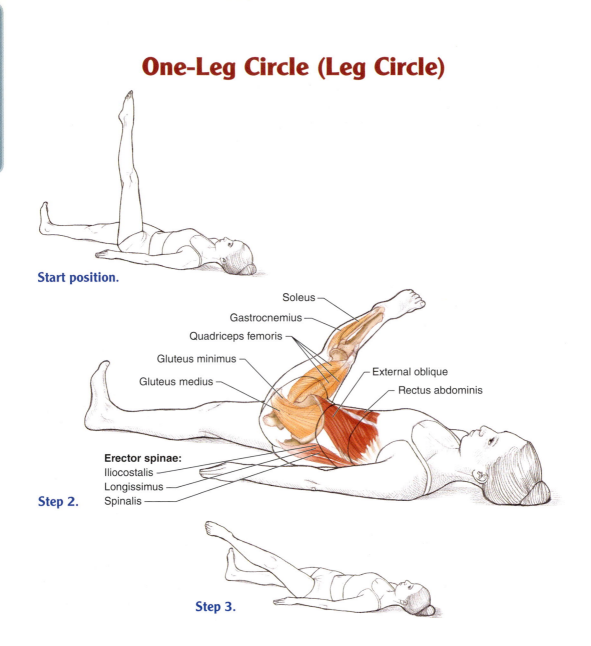

Start position.

Soleus
Gastrocnemius
Quadriceps femoris
Gluteus minimus
Gluteus medius
External oblique
Rectus abdominis
Erector spinae:
Iliocostalis
Longissimus
Spinalis

Step 2.

Step 3.

Execution

1. *Start position.* Lie supine with the arms by the sides and the palms facing down, both legs outstretched on the mat. Bend one knee to the chest, and straighten that leg toward the ceiling so that it is perpendicular to the mat. Gently point the foot. Flex the foot on the mat (ankle–foot dorsiflexion).

2. *Exhale.* Circle the raised leg across the midline of the body, allowing one side of the pelvis to lift off the mat. See the main muscle illustration. Continue to circle the leg down and across the other leg as the back of the pelvis returns to lie evenly on the mat.

3. *Inhale.* Continue to circle the leg out to the same side as it was originally raised to return to the start position. Repeat the same pattern with the other leg, alternating the legs with each circle. Do five circles with each leg.

Targeted Muscles

Anterior spinal rotators and stabilizers: rectus abdominis, external oblique, internal oblique, transversus abdominis

Posterior spinal rotators and stabilizers: erector spinae (iliocostalis, longissimus, spinalis), semispinalis, deep posterior spinal group

Accompanying Muscles

Hip flexors: iliopsoas, rectus femoris

Hip extensors: gluteus maximus, hamstrings

Hip abductors: gluteus medius, gluteus minimus

Hip adductors: adductor longus, adductor brevis, adductor magnus, gracilis

Knee extensors: quadriceps femoris

Ankle–foot plantar flexors: gastrocnemius, soleus

Ankle–foot dorsiflexors: tibialis anterior, extensor digitorum longus

Technique Cues

- In step 1, think of pulling up the front and back of the pelvis simultaneously so that this cocontraction of the abdominals and spinal extensors can be used to limit an excessive anterior or posterior pelvic tilt while the spinal rotators allow the pelvis to rotate carefully from side to side to complement the leg's circling movements.

- Maintain a long line with the circling leg by using the knee extensors to keep the knee straight and the ankle–foot plantar flexors to maintain a pointed position of the raised foot. The ankle–foot dorsiflexors maintain a flexed position of the foot on the mat.

- Focus on using the hip muscles in a finely coordinated manner to create a smooth leg circle. For example, in step 2 use the hip adductors initially to bring the leg across the body and the hip extensors to produce the down part of the circle. The hip abductors then quickly become active to prevent the leg from dropping too far toward the mat. In step 3, the hip flexors are key in producing the up portion of the circle, while the hip abductors also work initially to bring the leg to the side.

- While keeping the movement smooth, add an emphasis at the end of each circle as the leg returns to its vertical position, pausing momentarily.

- *Imagine.* Imagine a string from the ceiling guiding your leg in a circular motion, like a string puppet. At the same time, your pelvis and spine roll from center to side and back like a pendulum. The sideways pendulum movement and the circular leg motion are coordinated perfectly to provide a smooth, uninterrupted flow of movement.

(continued)

Exercise Notes

Although many hip muscles are used in One-Leg Circle, the resistance is insufficient to offer much strength benefit for these muscles. Instead, this exercise offers the benefit of hip mobility, including a dynamic stretch for the hamstrings. In some cases, it can help relieve muscle tightness or spasm in the hip and lower back. In addition, this exercise teaches the complex skill of moving the leg in many directions while controlling the accompanying pelvic movement. For example, as the leg moves down, the tendency is for the pelvis to tilt anteriorly and the lower back to arch. Firm contraction of the abdominals as if to create a posterior pelvic tilt is required to counter this tendency. Similarly, as the leg moves across the body or out to the side, the spinal rotators must first contract to start the pelvic rotation and then work in the opposite manner as if to counterrotate the pelvis to prevent the pelvis from rotating excessively in the direction of the circling leg. Lastly, as the leg comes back to vertical, slight simultaneous contraction of the back extensors with the abdominals is often required to prevent the pelvis from posteriorly tilting.

Variations

A common variation is to circle the leg 5 to 10 times in one direction and then the other direction before switching legs. The exercise can also be performed with the arms out at shoulder height (T position), palms facing up. This variation provides more stability and is beneficial when rolled shoulders are present. Also, reversing the position of the feet so the raised foot is flexed (ankle–foot dorsiflexion) can accentuate the dynamic hamstring stretch for the circling leg. In addition, the pelvis and spine can be kept absolutely still throughout, adding a challenge in terms of pelvic–spinal stabilization. Finally, to lengthen the breath, inhale for one circle and exhale for one circle.

Roll-Up

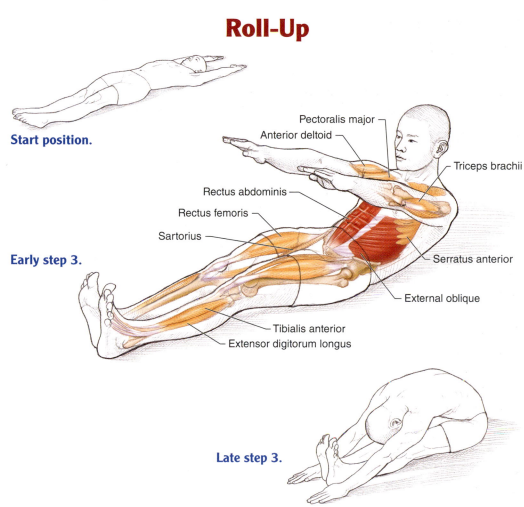

Start position.

Pectoralis major

Anterior deltoid

Triceps brachii

Rectus abdominis

Rectus femoris

Sartorius

Early step 3.

Serratus anterior

External oblique

Tibialis anterior

Extensor digitorum longus

Late step 3.

Execution

1. *Start position.* Lie supine, legs straight and together with the feet gently pointed. Arms are straight overhead and in line with the shoulders, palms facing up.

2. *Inhale.* After drawing the abdominal wall inward toward the spine, lift the arms toward the ceiling and bring the chin toward the chest while lifting the head and scapulae off the mat. Simultaneously flex the feet (ankle–foot dorsiflexion).

3. *Exhale.* Continue to curl up (see the main muscle illustration), passing through a sitting position until the upper body is over the legs, with the fingers reaching toward the toes. If flexibility allows, the palms can touch the sides of the feet or be placed on the mat as shown.

4. *Inhale.* Begin to roll down until the back of the sacrum starts to establish contact with the mat.

5. *Exhale.* Finish rolling down and then bring the arms overhead, returning to the start position. Repeat the sequence 10 times.

(continued)

Targeted Muscles

Spinal flexors: rectus abdominis, external oblique, internal oblique

Accompanying Muscles

Anterior spinal stabilizer: transversus abdominis

Spinal extensors: erector spinae

Hip flexors: iliopsoas, rectus femoris

Hip extensors: gluteus maximus, hamstrings

Ankle–foot dorsiflexors: tibialis anterior, extensor digitorum longus

Shoulder flexors: anterior deltoid, pectoralis major (clavicular)

Shoulder extensors: latissimus dorsi, teres major, pectoralis major (sternal)

Scapular depressors: lower trapezius, serratus anterior (lower fibers)

Elbow extensors: triceps brachii

Technique Cues

- Focus on a smooth, sequential movement of every vertebra as each one lifts off in steps 2 and 3 and lowers onto the mat in steps 4 and 5.
- Late in step 3, emphasize pulling the lower abdominals in while the hip extensors and spinal extensors smoothly control the trunk as it lowers, and the head, hands, and heels reach away from the center. Keep the head between the arms and the heels in contact with the mat as the fingers reach toward the toes.
- Focus on creating a long line with the arms by using the elbow extensors to keep the elbows straight and the scapular depressors to avoid elevating the scapulae toward your ears. Maintain this positioning of the arms as they move at the shoulder joints, with the shoulder extensors bringing the arms forward in step 2, the shoulder flexors preventing gravity from making the arms drop toward the mat in steps 3 and 4, and then the shoulder flexors starting to bring the arms overhead in step 5.
- *Imagine.* Pull the lower rib cage down and back. Imagine curling around a large exercise ball so the contraction of the abdominals keeps the back from flattening or arching as the hip flexors become more active and the trunk curls higher in step 3 and begins to lower in step 4.

Exercise Notes

Roll-Up challenges the abdominals and works on spinal articulation while the legs are straight instead of bent. This straight-leg position makes it more difficult for some people to achieve the posterior pelvic tilt and lower spine flexion that naturally accompany rolling up from a supine position. The straight-leg end position also offers a potential benefit of improving hamstring and lower back flexibility.

Modifications

If you are unable to come to a sitting position with good form, place small cuffs (maximum of 3 pounds [1.5 kg] each) on the ankles, or bend the knees slightly and use the hands (placed on the thighs) to help lift the upper trunk during the difficult part of the up phase.

Variation

This exercise can be performed with the feet gently pointed, the palms facing toward each other. Stop earlier with the shoulders over the hips as shown.

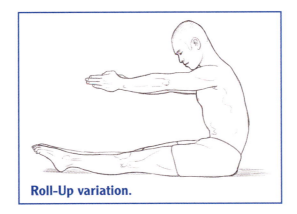

Roll-Up variation.

Neck Pull

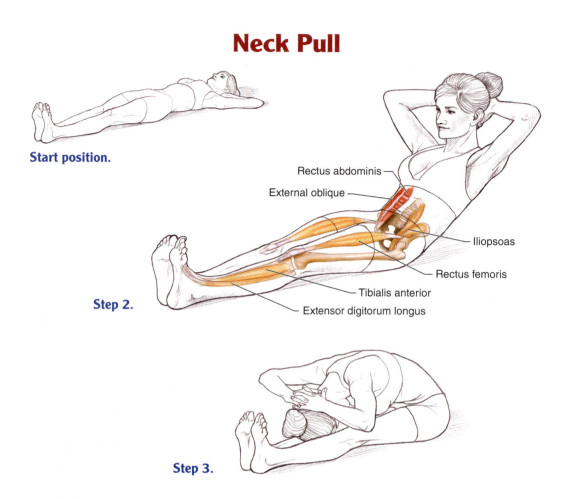

Start position.

Rectus abdominis

External oblique

Iliopsoas

Rectus femoris

Tibialis anterior

Extensor digitorum longus

Step 2.

Step 3.

Execution

1. *Start position.* Lie supine with the legs straight and together while the feet are flexed (ankle–foot dorsiflexion). The elbows are bent and out to the sides with the fingers interlaced behind the head.

2. *Inhale.* After drawing the abdominal wall inward toward the spine, bring the chin toward the chest while lifting the head and upper trunk off the mat. See the main muscle illustration.

3. *Exhale.* Continue to curl up through a sitting position until your upper body is rounded forward over your legs as shown.

4. *Inhale.* Begin rolling back in the rounded C-curve position.

5. *Exhale.* Complete rolling down to the start position. Repeat the sequence 10 times.

Targeted Muscles

Spinal flexors: rectus abdominis, external oblique, internal oblique

Accompanying Muscles

Anterior spinal stabilizer: transversus abdominis

Spinal extensors: erector spinae

Hip flexors: iliopsoas, rectus femoris

Hip extensors: gluteus maximus, hamstrings

Ankle–foot dorsiflexors: tibialis anterior, extensor digitorum longus

Technique Cues

- Focus on using the abdominals to create a smooth, sequential movement of each vertebra on the way up and on the way down.
- Think of using the abdominals to pull the front of the lower rib cage down and back to maximize flexion of the spine as you curl up to prevent the lower back from flattening or arching as the hip flexors become more active in step 3.
- As the upper body moves forward at the end of step 3, create a smooth, controlled movement through eccentric contraction of the hip extensors and back extensors, followed by the concentric use of these muscles to lift the trunk early in step 4.
- Contract the abdominals more intensely to maintain the C curve of the spine as long as possible while the abdominals help control lowering the trunk in step 5.
- Throughout the movement, keep the elbows reaching out to the sides as much as your strength allows. Don't jerk the elbows forward to aid the body during the curl-up. Despite the name of the exercise, avoid pulling on your head.
- *Imagine.* To achieve the desired quality of the movement, think of a wave building, cresting, and beginning to break as your trunk curls up in steps 1 through 3, a blowhole of water lifting your spine in step 4, and the tide pulling you back out to the sea as you lower your trunk in step 5.

Exercise Notes

Neck Pull shares many of the benefits of Roll-Up (page 73) but offers more challenge for abdominal strength because having the hands behind the head produces greater effective resistance (torque), as described in chapter 3. Developing skill in fine articulation of the lower back using this more difficult arm position is also valuable because this area of the spine is often tight, poorly controlled, and vulnerable to injury. This arm position provides a more rigorous dynamic stretch for the hamstrings and spinal extensors at the end of step 3.

Variations

Perform the first part of the exercise as described. However, instead of rolling back in the C-curve position from the point at which the trunk is over the legs, first roll up to a flat back position and sit upright. Then lean back on an angle, maintaining the flat back position before rounding the trunk and rolling all the way down to the start position. Neck Pull can also be performed with the feet gently pointed or flexed and the legs hip-width apart.

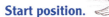

Hundred

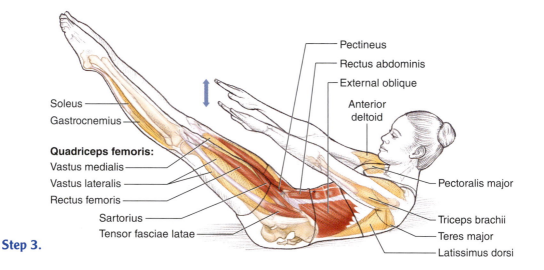

Start position.

Step 3.

Execution

1. *Start position.* Lie supine with the legs straight and raised about 60 degrees or higher, if necessary, to maintain pelvic stability. Gently point the feet. The arms rest on the mat beside the body, with the palms facing down.

2. *Exhale.* Draw the abdominal wall in, and lift the upper trunk into Chest Lift position (page 54). Bring the arms forward to 6 to 8 inches (15 to 20 cm) above the thighs, palms down.

3. *Inhale.* Pump the arms slightly down and then up on each count for a total of five counts with active breathing as described in chapter 1 (page 7). See the main muscle illustration.

4. *Exhale.* Pump the arms slightly down and then up on each count for a total of five counts with active breathing. Repeat this cycle 10 times or for 100 pumping motions, as long as good form can be maintained. Lower the torso and bring the arms back down to the start position.

Targeted Muscles

Spinal flexors: rectus abdominis, external oblique, internal oblique

Hip flexors: iliopsoas, rectus femoris, sartorius, tensor fasciae latae, pectineus

Accompanying Muscles

Anterior spinal stabilizer: transversus abdominis

Hip adductors: adductor longus, adductor brevis, adductor magnus, gracilis

Knee extensors: quadriceps femoris

Ankle–foot plantar flexors: gastrocnemius, soleus

Shoulder extensors: pectoralis major (sternal), latissimus dorsi, teres major

Shoulder flexors: pectoralis major (clavicular), anterior deltoid

Elbow extensors: triceps brachii

Technique Cues

- At the beginning of the exhale in step 2, draw the abdominal wall in toward the spine to encourage use of the transversus abdominis just before using the other abdominals to flex the spine, while at the start of the motion the shoulder flexors raise the arms.

- To achieve the desired end position in step 2, focus on maintaining a firm abdominal contraction so the lower back maintains contact with the mat and the pelvis remains stable. The hip flexors maintain the raised position of the legs, the knee extensors the straight position of the knees, and the ankle–foot plantar flexors the pointed position of the feet. Also, think of gently squeezing the inner thighs together to activate the hip adductors while reaching the legs out to create a long, arrowlike leg line.

- Maintain a stationary deep C curve of the trunk as the arms pump in steps 3 and 4.

- Use the elbow extensors to keep the elbows straight, and reach the fingertips forward.

- Focus on isolating the movement to the shoulder joints, trying to use the muscles that run just below the armpits to encourage activation of the large latissimus dorsi and pectoralis major as the shoulder extensors and flexors work together to produce the quick pumping movements of the arms.

- *Imagine.* Imagine you are pressing the arms down against a trampoline and they are rebounding a few inches.

(continued)

Hundred   *(continued)*

Exercise Notes

Hundred is one of the signature abdominal exercises of the Pilates repertoire. Hundred offers a particularly difficult challenge to core stability since you have to maintain a constant position of spinal flexion while holding your legs off the mat with the knees extended as the arms repetitively and vigorously move. Because of these challenges, Hundred benefits people with adequate strength and skill, but it is inappropriate and potentially high risk for people with inadequate strength or skill. Most people are not adequately prepared to perform this exercise with the legs held near to the mat. Use the modifications, and progress slowly to a more challenging leg position.

In Hundred, the contraction of the hip flexors holds the legs off the mat against gravity. As described in Leg Lift Supine (page 56), because of the attachments of the hip flexors (particularly the iliopsoas and rectus femoris) onto the spine and front of the pelvis, their contraction tends to cause the lower back to arch and the pelvis to tilt anteriorly unless adequate abdominal stabilization is performed simultaneously. (See the illustrations.) In Hundred, both legs are off the mat and the knees are straight. Therefore, the legs produce much greater torque, as described in chapter 3. This requires a much more forceful contraction of the hip flexors to keep the legs off the mat, and it is a greater challenge for the abdominals to stabilize the core and keep the lower back from arching. The closer the legs are to the mat, the greater the muscular force required to counter the weight of the legs.

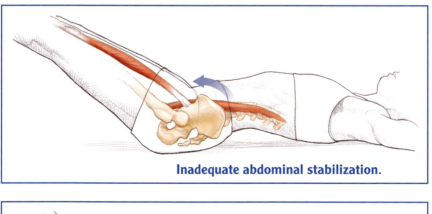

Inadequate abdominal stabilization.

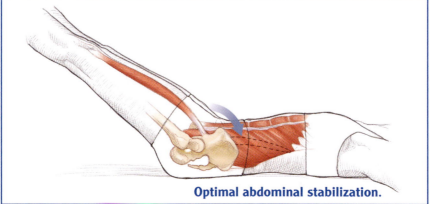

Optimal abdominal stabilization.

Modifications

Hold your legs as close to vertical as is necessary to allow you to maintain a stable pelvis and lower back. Gradually lower the legs as stability improves. If your hamstrings are tight, straighten the legs just until you feel tension in the hamstrings, or first practice the exercise with the legs in tabletop position or with the knees bent and the feet flat on the mat.

Variation

A variation on the breath pattern used in some approaches is to add a pause on the inhale in step 3 and then begin pumping the arms with the exhale. An exhale may make it easier to pull in the abdominal wall slightly farther to help establish firm pelvic stability as the arms pump for five counts. Once stability is established, try to maintain this position for the next five counts of the inhale and throughout the remainder of the 10 cycles.

One-Leg Stretch (Single-Leg Stretch)

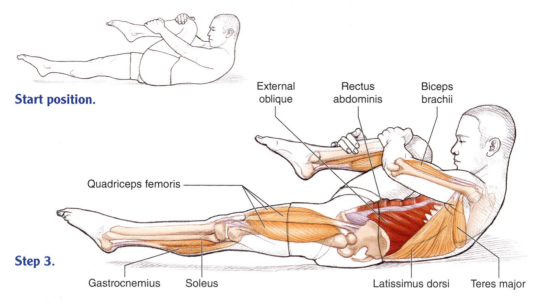

Start position.

External oblique

Rectus abdominis

Biceps brachii

Quadriceps femoris

Step 3.

Gastrocnemius   Soleus

Latissimus dorsi   Teres major

Execution

1. *Start position.* Lie supine with the head and scapulae off the mat in Chest Lift (page 54) position and one knee pulled into your chest. The hand on the side of the bent knee holds the shin just above the ankle. The other arm is bent with the hand on the knee. The straight leg is at a height at which the lower back can maintain contact with the mat. Both feet are gently pointed.

2. *Inhale.* Begin to bend the outstretched leg and straighten the bent leg.

3. *Exhale.* Complete the switch, using an exhale as the leg fully straightens and the hands switch to the other knee as shown in the main muscle illustration. The hand on the side of the bent knee grasps the shin near the ankle, and the other hand holds the knee that is pulled toward the chest. Repeat the sequence 5 times on each leg for a total of 10 times, completing each switch of the legs with an exhale.

Targeted Muscles

Spinal flexors: rectus abdominis, external oblique, internal oblique

Accompanying Muscles

Anterior spinal stabilizer: transversus abdominis

Hip flexors: iliopsoas, rectus femoris

Hip extensors: gluteus maximus, hamstrings

Knee extensors: quadriceps femoris

Ankle–foot plantar flexors: gastrocnemius, soleus

Shoulder flexors: anterior deltoid, pectoralis major (clavicular)

Shoulder extensors: latissimus dorsi, teres major, pectoralis major (sternal)

Elbow flexors: biceps brachii, brachialis

Elbow extensors: triceps brachii

Technique Cues

- In step 1, firmly pull the abdominal wall toward the spine. Maintain solid contact of the lower back and sacrum with the mat and a stationary position of the ASIS as you use the hip flexors and extensors to switch the legs in steps 2 and 3.
- Think of constantly lifting the upper trunk up and forward off the mat with a firm contraction of the abdominals so that it stays lifted at the same height instead of dropping down as the legs switch.
- While maintaining this core stability, reach one leg out in space. The knee extensors that straighten the knee and the ankle–foot plantar flexors that point the foot help to create the desired long line.
- Keep the scapulae neutral, and avoid lifting them toward your ears while the shoulder flexors work to keep the arms from dropping toward the mat when the arms switch to the opposite leg. The elbow extensors straighten the arm that reaches for the ankle, while the elbow flexors start bending the arm to bring it to the opposite knee. Use the elbow flexors on both arms to help pull the knee close to your chest. Then keep the knee stationary as the hands press down on the lower leg, and bring the elbows down toward the mat so that the shoulder extensors assist with keeping the torso lifted off the mat.
- *Imagine.* Imagine that your legs are moving precisely like pistons while the engine, the powerhouse of your body, remains entirely stationary.

Exercise Notes

One-Leg Stretch is a valuable stability exercise that emphasizes the abdominals. The abdominals work in multiple roles to keep the trunk lifted, maintain contact between the lower back and the mat, and keep the abdominal wall pulled in. This abdominal action is necessary to maintain pelvic and spinal stability, which the vigorous movement of the legs can easily disrupt.

Variation

This exercise can also be performed with the thigh of the bent leg just beyond vertical rather than close into the chest. Both hands are on that knee, with the lower part of the bent leg parallel to the mat. This alternative position can be used to emphasize curling up the trunk higher to better challenge the abdominals.

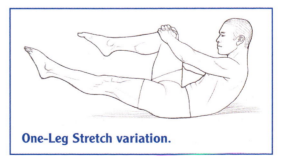

One-Leg Stretch variation.

Single Straight-Leg Stretch (Hamstring Pull)

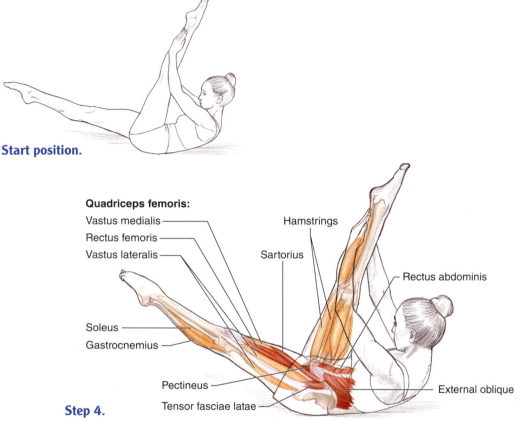

Start position.

Quadriceps femoris:

Vastus medialis

Rectus femoris

Vastus lateralis

Hamstrings

Sartorius

Rectus abdominis

Soleus

Gastrocnemius

Pectineus

External oblique

Tensor fasciae latae

Step 4.

Execution

1. *Start position.* Lie supine with the head and scapulae off the mat in Chest Lift (page 54) position. One leg is lifted toward the forehead, with both hands grasping it near the ankle. The opposite leg is suspended above the mat at a height at which the lower back can maintain contact with the mat. Both knees are straight and both feet are gently pointed.

2. *Exhale.* Pull the abdominal wall in slightly closer toward the spine while pulling the top leg closer to the forehead with two gentle pulses coordinated with two percussive exhales.

3. *Inhale.* While keeping the legs straight, switch the legs and move the hands to the ankle of the opposite leg.

4. *Exhale.* Again, pull this leg closer toward the forehead as shown in the main muscle illustration, with one percussive breath for each of the two pulses. Repeat the sequence 5 times on each leg, for a total of 10 times, switching the legs on the inhale and then pulling the top leg closer for two pulses with a double percussive exhale. When finished, return to the start position.

Targeted Muscles

Spinal flexors: rectus abdominis, external oblique, internal oblique

Hip flexors: iliopsoas, rectus femoris, sartorius, tensor fasciae latae, pectineus

Accompanying Muscles

Anterior spinal stabilizer: transversus abdominis

Hip extensors: gluteus maximus, hamstrings

Knee extensors: quadriceps femoris

Ankle–foot plantar flexors: gastrocnemius, soleus

Shoulder flexors: anterior deltoid, pectoralis major (clavicular)

Technique Cues

- In step 1, firmly pull the abdominal wall in toward the spine, and use a strong isometric abdominal contraction to keep the trunk lifted and the pelvis stable while maintaining contact between the lower back and the mat throughout the exercise, particularly as the legs switch.
- While maintaining core stability, reach both legs out in space. The knee extensors that straighten the knees and the ankle–foot plantar flexors that point the feet help to create the desired long line.
- Early in step 3, maintain the long leg line as you use the hip flexors to raise the lower leg and the hip extensors to lower the upper leg. After the upper leg passes vertical, the hip flexors become key in controlling it as it lowers against gravity.
- In step 4, focus on keeping this leg (now the lower leg) at a constant height as the top leg is gently pulled in toward the forehead. This creates a dynamic stretch for the hamstrings. Draw the top leg in using the shoulder flexors, with the elbows pointing to the sides.
- Concentrate on keeping the scapulae neutral rather than rounding forward or lifting up.
- *Imagine.* The leg switch should have a brisk and sharp dynamic, like opening and closing scissors, with the motion isolated to the hips.

Exercise Notes

As its name suggests, Single Straight-Leg Stretch is closely related to One-Leg Stretch (page 82), only both legs remain straight in Single Straight-Leg Stretch. Keeping the upper leg straight while bringing it toward the chest adds a beneficial dynamic stretch for the hamstrings, which often are tight. Lowering a straight leg requires more rigorous contraction of the abdominals to maintain stability of the pelvis and lower back.

(continued)

Single Straight-Leg Stretch (Hamstring Pull)   *(continued)*

Modifications

If the hamstrings are tight, move the hands lower on the leg, or allow the knee to bend slightly as the top leg is brought toward the forehead.

Variation

This exercise can be performed with the bottom leg lowered all the way to the mat as shown. This position can limit the posterior tilting of the pelvis, enhancing the stretch of the hamstrings on the top leg.

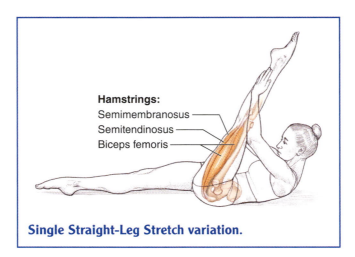

Hamstrings:
Semimembranosus
Semitendinosus
Biceps femoris

Single Straight-Leg Stretch variation.

Double-Leg Stretch

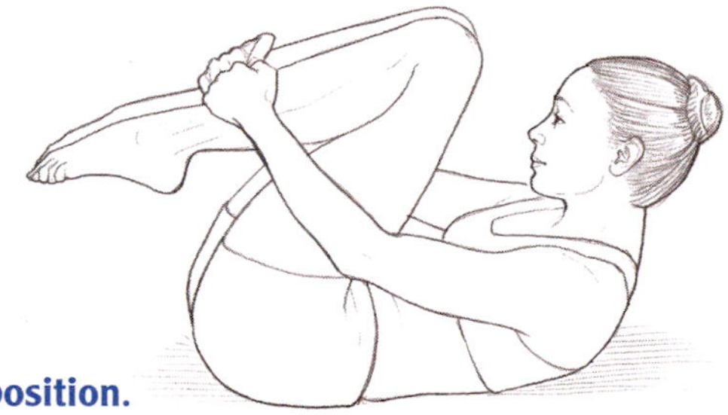

Start position.

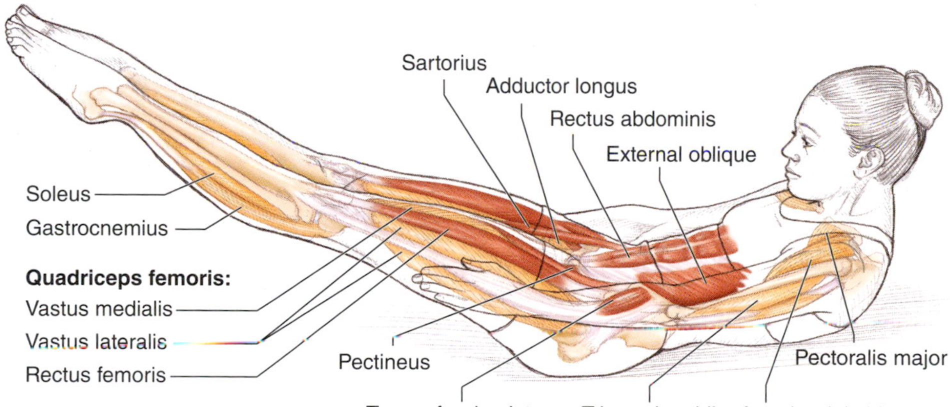

Step 2.

Sartorius
Adductor longus
Rectus abdominis
External oblique
Soleus
Gastrocnemius
Quadriceps femoris:
Vastus medialis
Vastus lateralis
Rectus femoris
Pectineus
Tensor fasciae latae
Triceps brachii
Anterior deltoid
Pectoralis major

Execution

1. *Start position.* Lie supine with the head and scapulae off the mat in Chest Lift (page 54) position, both knees bent and pulled toward the chest with one hand on each shin.

2. *Inhale.* Reach the arms down to the sides of the legs while simultaneously extending both legs to a height at which the lower back maintains contact with the mat. See the main muscle illustration.

3. *Exhale.* Bend the legs back in toward the chest while the arms return to the start position with the hands on the shins. Repeat the sequence 10 times.

Targeted Muscles

Spinal flexors: rectus abdominis, external oblique, internal oblique

Hip flexors: iliopsoas, rectus femoris, sartorius, tensor fasciae latae, pectineus

(continued)

Double-Leg Stretch   *(continued)*

Accompanying Muscles

Anterior spinal stabilizer: transversus abdominis

Hip extensors: gluteus maximus, hamstrings

Hip adductors: adductor longus, adductor brevis, adductor magnus, gracilis

Knee extensors: quadriceps femoris

Ankle–foot plantar flexors: gastrocnemius, soleus

Knee flexors: hamstrings

Shoulder flexors: anterior deltoid, pectoralis major (clavicular)

Elbow flexors: biceps brachii, brachialis

Elbow extensors: triceps brachii

Technique Cues

- In step 1, think of pulling together the lower attachments of the abdominals on the pelvis and the upper attachments on the rib cage and pulling the abdominal wall in to create a slight C curve. Maintain contact of the lower back with the mat throughout the exercise.

- While maintaining a curled stationary position of the trunk, reach both legs out. Use the hip extensors to begin to move the thighs away from the chest. The hip flexors then become key in supporting the weight of the legs and keeping the legs from lowering too far because of gravity. Gently pulling the legs together with the hip adductors as the knee extensors straighten the legs and the ankle–foot plantar flexors point the feet can help achieve the desired long leg line in step 2, before the hip flexors and knee flexors draw the legs in during step 3.

- As the arms move, think of reaching them toward the feet as the elbow extensors straighten the elbows in step 2. The elbow flexors bend the elbows in step 3. Throughout the exercise, the shoulder flexors keep the arms from lowering toward the mat because of gravity.

- *Imagine.* The movement should have a dynamic reach-and-gather quality, as if the limbs were springs being extended on the reach phase and then recoiling on the gather phase.

Exercise Notes

Double-Leg Stretch represents a large jump in difficulty from One-Leg Stretch (page 82). In the outstretched position, both legs are held far away from the axis of the motion, requiring abdominal strength and skill to maintain the desired core stability. While providing a valuable challenge for some, similar to that described for Hundred (page 78), this exercise is not appropriate for many individuals. Use modifications when needed.

Modifications

Straighten the legs to an angle as close to vertical as is necessary to allow the pelvis to remain stable and to avoid arching the lower back. If hamstring tightness is a limiting factor, the legs can be only partially straightened.

Variations

To challenge the abdominals more, reach the arms overhead as shown and then circle them around to the start position as the legs reach out and then come back in. Challenge the abdominals even more by keeping the thighs just beyond vertical when the knees bend and by curling the trunk up higher as described in One-Leg Stretch variation (page 83).

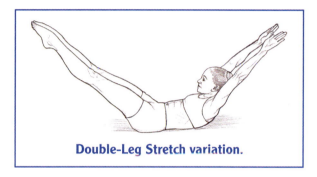

Double-Leg Stretch variation.

Crisscross

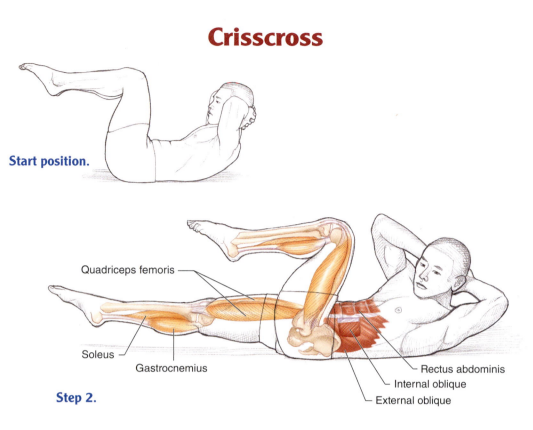

Start position.

Quadriceps femoris

Soleus

Gastrocnemius

Step 2.

Rectus abdominis
Internal oblique
External oblique

Execution

1. *Start position.* Lie supine with the head and scapulae off the mat in Chest Lift (page 54) position. Legs are in tabletop position but with knees slightly closer to the chest and both feet gently pointed. Arms are bent with the elbows out to the sides and the fingers interlaced behind the head.

2. *Exhale.* Straighten one leg while simultaneously rotating the trunk toward the opposite bent knee as shown in the main muscle illustration.

3. *Inhale.* Begin to straighten the bent leg and bend the straight leg while the upper torso rotates back to center.

4. *Exhale.* While switching the legs, rotate the trunk toward the opposite side. Fully straighten the one leg and bend the other toward the chest. Repeat the sequence 5 times on each leg for a total of 10 times, completing each switch of the legs and rotation of the upper trunk with a percussive exhale.

Targeted Muscles

Spinal flexors and rotators: rectus abdominis, external oblique, internal oblique, transversus abdominis

Accompanying Muscles

Hip flexors: iliopsoas, rectus femoris

Hip extensors: gluteus maximus, hamstrings

Knee extensors: quadriceps femoris

Ankle–foot plantar flexors: gastrocnemius, soleus

Technique Cues

- As described for the closely related One-Leg Stretch (page 82), firmly pull the abdominal wall in toward the spine in step 1, and maintain solid contact of the lower back and sacrum with the mat throughout the exercise.
- As the obliques, and potentially the transversus abdominis, rotate the upper trunk, keep the opposite side of the pelvis back so the pelvis doesn't rock in the direction of the rotation. Maintain even contact of the pelvis with the mat.
- Use the abdominals to maintain a C curve so that the upper trunk stays lifted as it rotates.
- While maintaining core stability, dynamically reach out one leg, with the hip extensors initially acting to take the thigh away from the chest. Optimally use the knee extensors that straighten the knee and the ankle–foot plantar flexors that point the foot to achieve the desired long leg line.
- Keep the scapulae neutral, and avoid lifting them up toward your ears.
- *Imagine.* Think of reaching the leg out in space as if a string were attached to the toe, pulling it out to coordinate the use of the hip flexors toward the end of the reach. The hip flexors keep the leg from falling to the mat because of gravity and then begin to bring the outstretched leg up toward the chest during the switch in step 3.

Exercise Notes

Crisscross is closely related to One-Leg Stretch (page 82) but potentially offers a greater challenge to the abdominals because of the more difficult position of the hands behind the head. Furthermore, the rotation adds more multiplane stability challenges and greater work for the obliques and transversus abdominis. These muscles are key for stabilizing the spine before movement of the limbs or before impact in activities such as lifting objects, running, and jumping.

Recruitment of the obliques and transversus abdominis requires fine-tuned technique. As described in Chest Lift With Rotation (page 64), maintaining the C curve while bringing one side of the rib cage toward the opposite hip can help with the desired activation. Also try to rotate around a central axis without letting the rib cage shift to one side relative to the central axis or bend toward one side of the pelvis (spinal lateral flexion), a common mistake.

Teaser

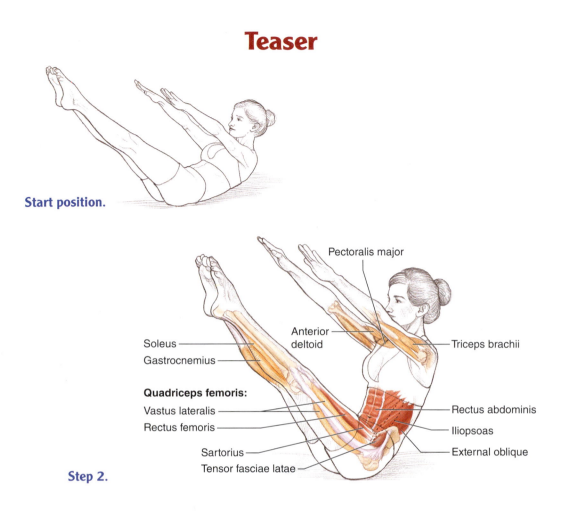

Start position.

Pectoralis major

Soleus

Anterior deltoid

Triceps brachii

Gastrocnemius

Quadriceps femoris:

Vastus lateralis

Rectus abdominis

Rectus femoris

Iliopsoas

Sartorius

External oblique

Tensor fasciae latae

Step 2.

Execution

1. *Start position.* Lie supine with the head and scapulae lifted off the mat and the abdominal wall drawn in toward the spine. Hold the legs together approximately 60 degrees off the mat, if stability can be maintained, with the knees straight and feet pointed. Reach forward with the arms, palms down, so the hands are parallel to the legs.

2. *Inhale.* Curl the upper trunk forward and upward until the body is balanced on the buttocks as shown in the main muscle illustration. Keep arms parallel to the legs.

3. *Exhale.* Curl the trunk back down to the start position. Repeat the sequence five times.

Targeted Muscles

Spinal flexors: rectus abdominis, external oblique, internal oblique

Hip flexors: iliopsoas, rectus femoris, sartorius, tensor fasciae latae, pectineus

Accompanying Muscles

Anterior spinal stabilizer: transversus abdominis

Hip adductors: adductor longus, adductor brevis, adductor magnus, gracilis

Knee extensors: quadriceps femoris

Ankle–foot plantar flexors: gastrocnemius, soleus

Shoulder flexors: anterior deltoid, pectoralis major (clavicular)

Elbow extensors: triceps brachii

Technique Cues

- Focus on pulling the abdominal wall in firmly to prevent the lower back from arching or the pelvis from tilting anteriorly as the hip flexors, particularly the iliopsoas, contract forcibly to hold the legs in the air, especially when the hip flexors are helping raise and lower the torso in the upper movement ranges of steps 2 and 3.
- Keep the legs stationary throughout the exercise. Use the hip adductors to pull the legs together slightly as you reach them out in space, with the knee extensors keeping the knees straight and the ankle–foot plantar flexors pointing the feet.
- Focus on using the abdominals to achieve a smooth, sequential movement as each vertebra lifts off the mat, from the top of the spine to the bottom in step 2 and from the bottom of the spine to the top in step 3. Avoid hinging from the hips, which is evidence of excessive use of the hip flexors.
- Focus on creating a long arm line by using the elbow extensors to keep the elbows straight. At the same time, avoid elevating the scapulae toward your ears by using the scapular depressors as the shoulder flexors work to keep the arms appropriately positioned in front of the body.
- Move the arms in accordance with the legs to maintain a parallel relationship.
- *Imagine.* Imagine that someone is lightly holding your toes, so that the legs remain entirely stationary, as you raise and lower the trunk only.

(continued)

Teaser   *(continued)*

Exercise Notes

Teaser is a signature Pilates exercise that builds abdominal and hip flexor strength and endurance while incorporating skilled spinal articulation and keen balance. It combines the fine articulation of the spine used in Roll-Up (page 73) with the legs off the mat practiced in Hundred (page 78) and Double-Leg Stretch (page 87). Also, Rocker With Open Legs (page 108) can be very helpful in practicing the balance required. If the torso is raised too high for your current hamstring flexibility, the body will tend to fall forward. If the legs are raised too high for your current hamstring flexibility and abdominal strength, the trunk will tend to fall backward. A skilled counterbalance of body segments and coordinated coactivation of abdominal and hip flexors are essential for successful execution of this form of Teaser.

Teaser was put at the end of this chapter because it requires a synthesis of many components of skills practiced with prior exercises. If inadequate strength or skill prevents optimal form, use modifications until you develop the necessary components. The weight of the legs is great, and inadequate stabilization of the pelvis and lower back can produce lower back strain or injury. Furthermore, this exercise is considered high risk by some people in the medical community and should not be performed if you experience any back discomfort or if it is contraindicated for you for any reason.

Modification

If you are having trouble smoothly rolling up to a high V position, bend the knees slightly. This slackens the hamstrings to allow a higher position of the torso and reduces the difficulty by bringing the legs closer to the pelvis so that the effect of the weight of the legs is reduced (less torque).

Variations

There are many variations for this exercise. Some schools call the exercise described here, or similar versions in which the legs stay stationary and only the trunk moves, Teaser 1. Teaser 2 involves maintaining the trunk in the lifted position while raising and lowering only the legs. Teaser 3 involves lowering both the legs and trunk simultaneously toward the mat and then lifting both simultaneously to the V position.

Many schools of Pilates training also use upper back extension, rather than a flexed spine, in the V position. This adds a valuable countermeasure for slumped posture (kyphosis) as well as practice of cocontracting the abdominals so the spinal extensors create the desired extension of the thoracic spine without creating undesired hyperextension of the lumbar spine. This variation also may incorporate bringing the arms to an overhead position while in the V position as shown and when the torso is in its low position at the end of step 3.

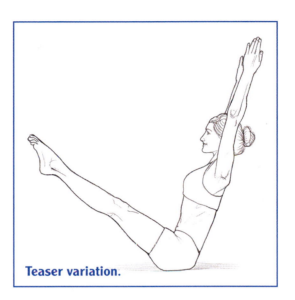

Teaser variation.

FINE ARTICULATION
FOR A FLEXIBLE SPINE

Movement of the spine is a complex process. As previously described in chapter 2, the spine is made up of 24 movable vertebrae in the neck (cervical), upper back (thoracic), and lower back (lumbar) that are joined by cartilage discs at their bodies and small gliding joints in their arches. Numerous ligaments and muscles connect the vertebrae. The five fused vertebrae of the sacrum move as a unit relative to the lowest lumbar vertebra.

A goal of Pilates is to achieve precise, sequential movement of each vertebra relative to the next vertebra. The desired precise movement is called *spinal articulation.* In anatomy, articulation simply refers to a joint, but other usages, such as "to utter distinctly each note in a musical phrase" or "the action or manner of jointing or interrelating," are more akin to its use in Pilates. The term *fine articulation* clarifies that one aim of the exercises in this chapter is to promote finely coordinated spinal movements.

The spine moves in many directions, and the goal of Pilates is to achieve finely coordinated movements in all directions. Of particular importance is spinal flexion, this chapter's focus. Many people lack flexibility in their lower backs and have difficulty achieving normal motion. Because the lower back naturally arches backward (concave to the back), spinal flexion tends to open this curve and can help restore healthy flexibility. Other people may have adequate flexibility but lack fine control.

Since the abdominal muscles are spinal flexors, the exercises in chapter 5 and this chapter share many similarities and benefits. While the exercises in chapter 5 focused more on muscular strength and endurance, the exercises in this chapter emphasize spinal mobility and articulation. Spine Stretch (page 98) uses precise spinal flexion from a sitting position. The next four exercises require you to maintain a finely articulated spine in a fixed flexed position while rolling. Rolling Back (page 100) develops the basic skills, while Seal (page 102) increases the difficulty by adding quick leg movements. Crab (page 104) advances to include greater movement forward, up, and over the knees. Rocker With Open Legs (page 108) requires you to hold both legs in a V position while rolling. The next four exercises provide a strong hamstring and lower back stretch. Rollover With Legs Spread (page 112) introduces basic skills before Control Balance (page 120) adds lifting one leg and Jackknife (page 123) both legs from a flexed spine position. Boomerang (page 116) combines the skills of Rollover With Legs Spread with the balance challenges of Teaser (page 92).

This chapter contains some of the most controversial Pilates exercises, including some involving extreme spinal flexion in which the body weight is borne by the shoulders and neck. Although many practitioners proclaim the benefits of these exercises, many medical specialists warn of their risks. Take extra caution with these exercises. Seek medical counsel to see if these exercises or their modifications are appropriate for you. Adequately warm up before exercising, and do not progress to more advanced exercises until you have mastered the basic versions. Medical practitioners generally recommend that exercises that require bearing weight on the neck be avoided by pregnant women, peri- and postmenopausal women, and people with osteoporosis or neck problems. Some types of lower back problems can be aggravated by flexion, although others may be aided.

Spine Stretch (Spine Stretch Forward)

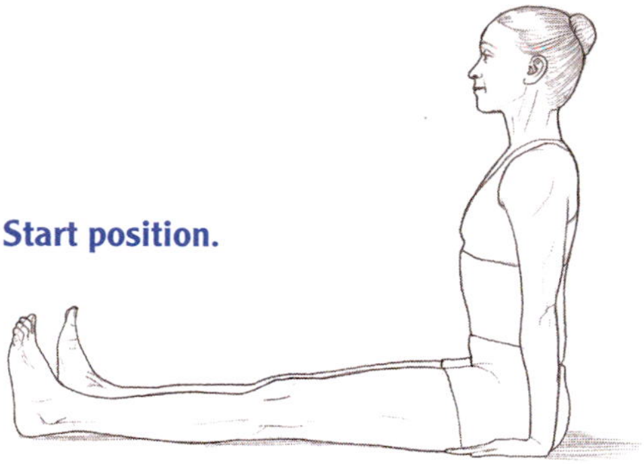

Start position.

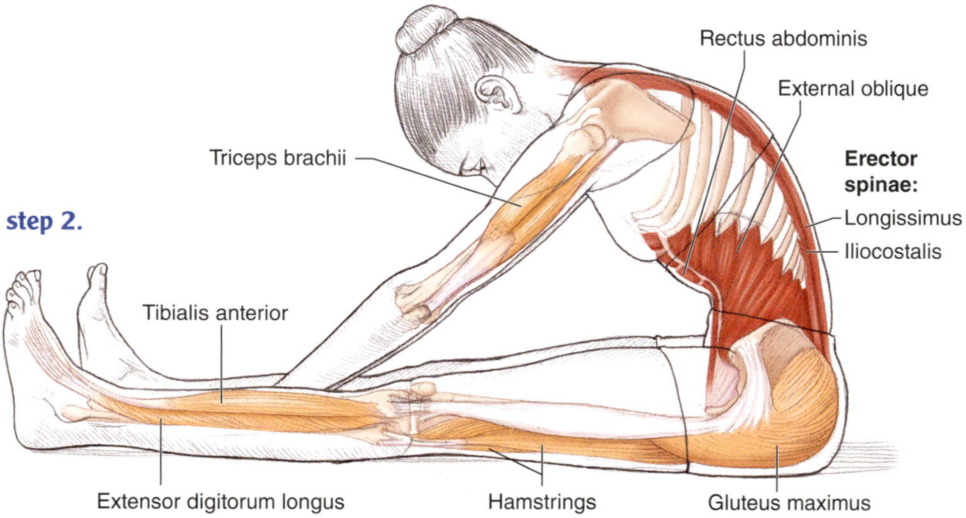

Early step 2.

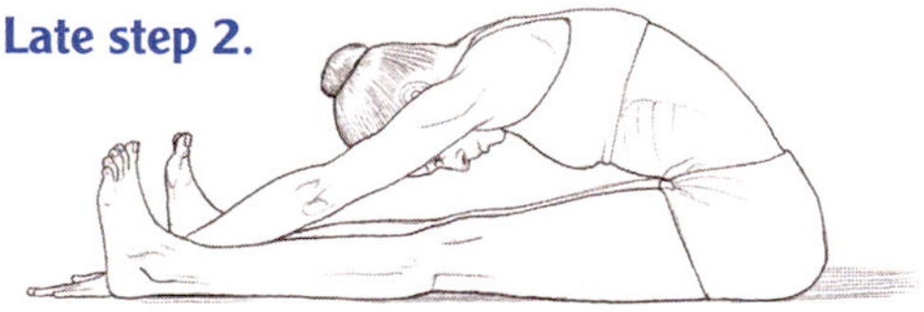

Rectus abdominis

External oblique

Triceps brachii

Erector spinae:

Longissimus

Iliocostalis

Tibialis anterior

Extensor digitorum longus

Hamstrings

Gluteus maximus

Late step 2.

Execution

1. *Start position.* Sit with the trunk upright. Knees are straight, legs slightly wider than shoulder-width apart, and feet flexed (ankle–foot dorsiflexion). Hold the arms straight by your sides with your palms on the mat.

2. *Exhale.* Draw the abdominal wall in as your head and upper spine roll down and your arms reach forward. See the main muscle illustration. Glide your hands across the mat on the insides of your legs as shown.

3. *Inhale.* Roll the spine back up, returning to the start position. Repeat the sequence five times.

Targeted Muscles

Spinal extensors: erector spinae (spinalis, longissimus, iliocostalis), semispinalis, deep posterior spinal group

Spinal flexors: rectus abdominis, external oblique, internal oblique

Accompanying Muscles

Anterior spinal stabilizer: transversus abdominis

Hip extensors: gluteus maximus, hamstrings

Ankle–foot dorsiflexors: tibialis anterior, extensor digitorum longus

Shoulder flexors: anterior deltoid, pectoralis major (clavicular)

Elbow extensors: triceps brachii

Technique Cues

- At the beginning of step 2, keep your head close to your trunk as you roll down. Use the abdominals both to pull the abdominal wall inward and to bring the front of the rib cage down and back to maximize spinal flexion in the sitting position. As the abdominals create this desired scooped shape of the lower trunk, use the spinal extensors to smoothly control the lowering of the upper trunk caused by gravity. Sequentially move down the spine one vertebra at a time.

- Initially focus on keeping the pelvis vertical, using an isometric contraction of the hip extensors to prevent the top of the pelvis from moving forward relative to the thighs (i.e., preventing hip flexion) as you begin to reach forward.

- At the end of step 2, tilt the top of the pelvis forward slightly, and reach the arms farther forward to maximize the hamstring stretch.

- Emphasize the reach of the legs by using the ankle–foot dorsiflexors to flex the feet. Focus on reaching the heels forward while keeping them in contact with the mat.

- To achieve the desired reach of the arms, keep the scapulae down in a neutral position while the shoulder flexors help slide the arms forward and the elbow extensors keep the elbows straight to create a sense of length.

- During the roll-up in step 3, use the abdominals to pull the abdominal wall in. Simultaneously think of stacking one vertebra at a time on the sacrum, this time from the lumbar spine up, as the spinal extensors bring the spine back to vertical.

- *Imagine.* During the roll-down and roll-up, imagine a strap around your waist being pulled from behind, deepening your scooped center, as your arms and legs reach forward.

Exercise Notes

Spine Stretch provides a perfect opportunity to practice detailed articulation of the spine from a stable sitting position using two key spinal positions, straight and rounded. A common goal in Pilates when flexing the spine is to emphasize rounding the lower back, not just the upper back. Because the upper back (thoracic spine) naturally is concave to the front, it is very easy to overexaggerate rounding forward in this portion of the spine. This exercise allows you to focus on achieving adequate rounding in the lower back and provides a dynamic stretch for the hamstrings and lower spinal extensors.

Rolling Back (Rolling Like a Ball)

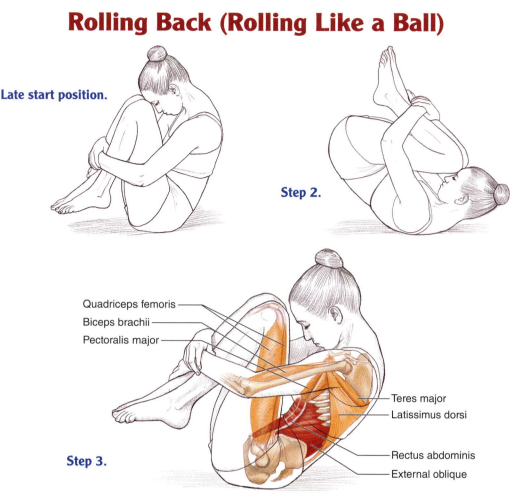

Late start position.

Step 2.

Quadriceps femoris

Biceps brachii

Pectoralis major

Teres major

Latissimus dorsi

Rectus abdominis

External oblique

Step 3.

Execution

1. *Start position.* Sit with your knees drawn close to your chest, legs together so your body is in a tight ball with your feet resting on the mat. Place your head as close to your knees as your flexibility allows. Firmly grasp your lower legs. Rock back on your sit bones so that you are balanced with your feet suspended slightly above the mat.
2. *Inhale.* Roll back onto your upper back as shown.
3. *Exhale.* Roll forward (as shown in the main muscle illustration) to return to the start position. Repeat the sequence 10 times.

Targeted Muscles

Spinal flexors and anterior stabilizers: rectus abdominis, external oblique, internal oblique, transversus abdominis

Accompanying Muscles

Hip flexors: iliopsoas, rectus femoris

Hip extensors: gluteus maximus, hamstrings

Hip adductors: adductor longus, adductor brevis, adductor magnus, gracilis

Knee extensors: quadriceps femoris

Shoulder extensors: latissimus dorsi, teres major, pectoralis major (sternal)

Elbow flexors: biceps brachii, brachialis

Technique Cues

- In step 1, scoop the abdominal wall in to create a deep C curve from the head to the coccyx. The hip flexors help hold the legs off the mat.
- At the beginning of step 2, pull in the lower abdominal wall even farther so that the ASIS and trunk roll back. Use just enough momentum to smoothly roll onto your upper back.
- To help reverse the direction of motion in step 3, think of using your hip extensors to bring your thighs away from your chest. (The arms will stop actual change in hip joint angle.) Use your shoulder extensors to pull your feet down. At the same time, use the abdominals to deepen lumbar flexion and raise the upper trunk to achieve the desired forward roll.
- Throughout the exercise, focus on minimizing the changes in the angles at the hips, knees, and elbows. Think of the body rolling as a whole. To help achieve this constant shape, balance isometric contractions of the arms and legs to maintain tension but no visible movement. Think of using the hip extensors to bring your knees slightly away from your body and the knee extensors to slightly extend the knees as your elbow flexors counter these potential motions by pulling the lower legs toward the buttocks.
- Use the hip adductors to keep the legs together as the body rolls.
- *Imagine.* Imagine you are on the inside of an exercise ball, maintaining a consistent curve of your spine against the arc of the ball as the ball rolls smoothly back and forth.

Exercise Notes

Rolling Back applies articulation of the spine in a different way. Here the goal is to maintain a constant flexed shape of the spine and contact each vertebra sequentially as the body rolls back and then forward in space. This requires shifting strategies for muscle activation and balance. This challenging skill will be used in many other exercises in this and later chapters.

Modification

If you are tight in the lower back or hips, have difficulty returning to the start position, or use too much movement of the lower legs, start with one hand on the back of each thigh just below the knee.

Variation

Place one hand just above each ankle, elbows pointing out, with the spine in a more gradual C curve, while emphasizing greater flexion in the lumbar region and less flexion in the upper back.

Seal (Seal Puppy)

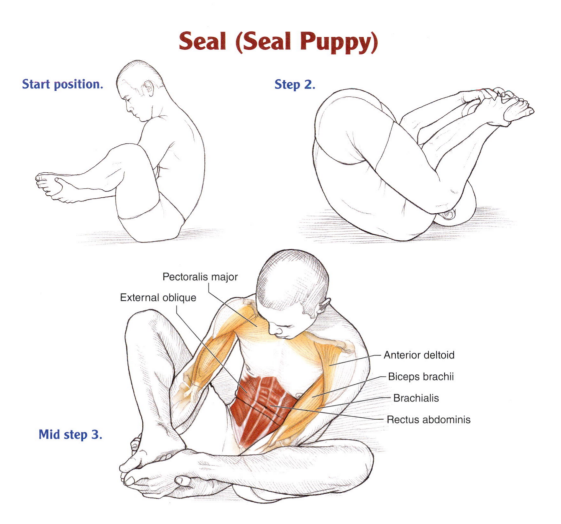

Start position.

Step 2.

Pectoralis major

External oblique

Anterior deltoid

Biceps brachii

Brachialis

Rectus abdominis

Mid step 3.

Execution

1. *Start position.* Sit with the knees bent toward the chest and open slightly beyond shoulder width, heels together, with the spine in a C curve. Bring the arms between the thighs and then under the lower legs so that each hand grasps the outside of the respective foot. Lift the feet off the mat, raising the knees to outside the shoulders. Rock back on the sit bones to balance.

2. *Inhale.* Roll back onto your upper back as shown.

3. *Exhale.* Roll forward to return to the start position as shown in the main muscle illustration. Clap the feet together twice. Repeat the sequence 10 times.

Targeted Muscles

Spinal flexors and anterior stabilizers: rectus abdominis, external oblique, internal oblique, transversus abdominis

Accompanying Muscles

Hip flexors: iliopsoas, rectus femoris

Hip abductors: gluteus medius, gluteus minimus

Hip adductors: adductor longus, adductor brevis, adductor magnus, gracilis

Knee extensors: quadriceps femoris

Shoulder flexors: anterior deltoid, pectoralis major (clavicular)

Elbow flexors: biceps brachii, brachialis

Technique Cues

- In step 1, use the abdominal muscles to create a posterior pelvic tilt and C curve from the head to the coccyx. At the same time, pull in the abdominal wall so the front side of the trunk is scooped inward toward the spine. Use the hip flexors to hold the legs off the mat and keep the thighs close to the chest. The shoulder flexors and elbow flexors also help the arms hold the legs close to the shoulders with the hips in an externally rotated position.

- At the beginning of step 2, pull in the lower abdominal wall even farther so the ASIS rotate backward and the body rolls back smoothly onto the upper back.

- To help reverse the direction of motion in step 3, use the hip extensors to bring your thighs away from your chest and your hands to pull your legs down. (The arms will stop actual change in hip joint angle.) At the same time, use the abdominals to deepen lumbar flexion and raise the upper trunk to achieve the desired forward roll of the body as a whole.

- As the body rolls, attempt to maintain a constant shape of the body, applying the concepts described here and in Rolling Back (page 100).

- Once you reach the balance start position, gently clap the feet together twice, using the hip abductors to open the legs and the hip adductors to close the legs. The emphasis is on the closing of the legs with a quick and sharp dynamic.

- *Imagine.* To achieve the desired smooth rolling of the body, imagine that your spine is the arc of a ball, wheel, or hoop that retains its curve as the object rolls.

Exercise Notes

Seal gets its name from the claps of the feet, likened to a seal clapping its flippers. Seal shares many of the benefits and challenges of Rolling Back (page 100), such as a dynamic stretch for the spinal extensors, coordinated use of the abdominals to maintain a C curve of the spine while rolling, skilled use of momentum, and the rock back on the sit bones to balance. In the top position, Seal adds the challenge of feet claps, which can easily disrupt momentum, balance, or maintenance of the C curve.

Modification

If lack of balance or flexibility limits your ability to perform Seal, begin with your knees farther from your shoulders, arms outside the upper thighs, and hands grasping the backs of the thighs just above the knees.

Variation

For an additional challenge, clap the feet three times at both the bottom and the top positions of the movement, pausing before rolling.

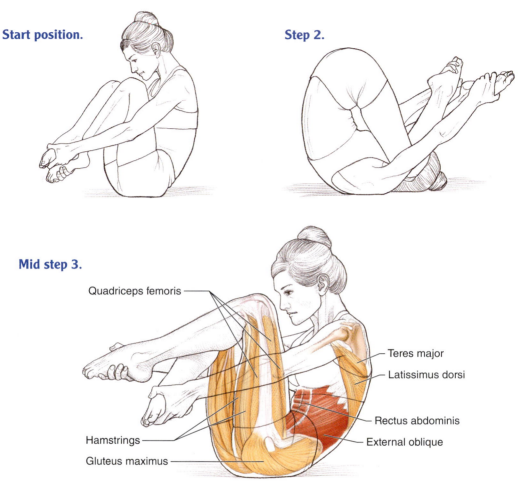

Crab

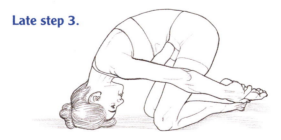

Start position.

Step 2.

Mid step 3.

Quadriceps femoris

Teres major

Latissimus dorsi

Rectus abdominis

External oblique

Hamstrings

Gluteus maximus

Late step 3.

Execution

1. *Start position.* Sit with your knees bent and one ankle crossed in front of the other. The spine is in a C curve. Bringing your arms around your thighs, grasp each foot with the opposite hand (left foot with right hand and right foot with left hand), elbows pointing out and slightly bent. Place the thumbs on the insides of the feet, fingers wrapping under the arches. Lift the feet off the mat, raising the knees inside the shoulders. Rock back on the sit bones to balance.

2. *Inhale.* Roll back onto your upper back as shown.

3. *Exhale.* Roll forward through the start position (see the main muscle illustration) to place the head on the mat as shown. Rolling back to the start position again, repeat the entire sequence six times. After the final repetition, return to the balance start position.

Targeted Muscles

Spinal flexors and anterior stabilizers: rectus abdominis, external oblique, internal oblique, transversus abdominis

Accompanying Muscles

Hip flexors: iliopsoas, rectus femoris

Hip extensors: gluteus maximus, hamstrings

Hip external rotators: gluteus maximus, deep outward rotators

Knee extensors: quadriceps femoris

Shoulder extensors: latissimus dorsi, teres major, pectoralis major (sternal)

Elbow flexors: biceps brachii, brachialis

Technique Cues

- In step 1, use the abdominal muscles to create a posterior pelvic tilt and C curve from the head to the coccyx. At the same time, pull in the abdominal wall so the front side of the trunk is scooped inward toward the spine. Use the hip flexors to hold the legs off the mat and keep the thighs close to the chest. The hips are externally rotated slightly so the knees go toward the insides of the shoulders.

- At the beginning of step 2, pull in the lower abdominal wall even farther so the ASIS rotate posteriorly and the body rolls smoothly onto the upper back. Try to minimize changes in the C curve of the spine and angles of flexion at the hips and knees.

(continued)

Crab *(continued)*

- To help reverse the direction of motion at the beginning of step 3, think of using the hip extensors to bring your thighs away from your chest and your shoulder extensors to pull the feet toward your buttocks. As described in Rolling Back (page 100), coordinated simultaneous contraction of the knee extensors and elbow flexors minimizes undesired changes in joint angles and facilitates the forward rolling of the body as a whole. Use the abdominals to deepen lumbar flexion as you begin the roll and then to bring the upper trunk up later in the rolling motion (mid step 3).

- As the body weight shifts over the knees in late step 3, think of lifting the pelvis up and over the knees through a combined contraction of the hip extensors, knee extensors, and abdominals. Here the angle of knee flexion decreases to allow the trunk to come forward so the head can touch the mat, while the hip external rotators act to maintain the same outward facing of the knees.

- In step 3 when the head is on the mat, carefully control the force and speed of the forward movement so that the forces applied to the small vertebrae of the neck remain very low.

- During the return to the start position, fine eccentric use of the knee extensors and hip extensors is important for controlling the lowering of the pelvis and protecting the knees.

- *Imagine.* During the challenging phase of rolling over the knees and placing the head on the mat, imagine a partner pulling up and forward on the belt loops of your jeans to lift your pelvis. Use this same image as you roll back. This may help you achieve the desired smooth, light, and lifted feel of the movement.

Exercise Notes

Crab may get its name from the similarity between the shape of the legs—knees to the sides and feet coming toward the center—used in this exercise and the shape of the front clawed appendages of a crab. Crab is an advanced exercise that should be attempted only by very skilled students of Pilates and only after Rolling Back (page 100) and Seal (page 102) can be performed with excellent form. It shares many of the benefits of these two exercises, including a dynamic stretch for the spinal extensors, coordinated use of the abdominals and other muscles to maintain the body in a ball shape as it rolls, skilled use of momentum, and sophisticated balance on a small base of support.

However, Crab adds a new challenge—forward movement of the body with the knees in a vulnerable position, deep knee flexion that is weight bearing. In addition, the knees point somewhat to the sides rather than straight ahead, making twisting of the knees a potential problem if good form is not applied. Furthermore, the end position stretches the neck in a way that could be dangerous if good control is not maintained. Therefore, it is wise that this exercise not be performed by people with knee problems, neck problems, or other conditions that could increase the potential risk of injury associated with it.

Variation

While performing Crab, uncross and recross the legs in the rolled-back position. The knees may either remain bent or straighten as shown and then bend again. This variation adds a fun challenge to Crab. The quick movements of the legs and arms require coordinated use of the many associated muscles to avoid disrupting core stability or the flow of the movement. This variation also uses a slightly different position of the hands that some people may find helps them keep a more neutral position of the feet. To allow time for careful inclusion of the new elements while keeping the exhale on the most difficult up phase of the movement, adjust the breath pattern. Exhale on the roll-back, inhale as the legs change, exhale on the roll-up, and inhale for the gentle neck stretch.

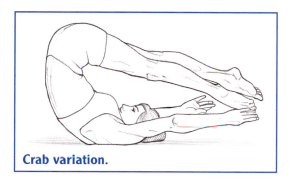

Crab variation.

Rocker With Open Legs
(Open-Leg Rocker)

Start position.

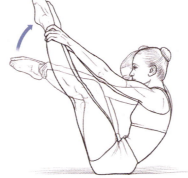

Step 2.

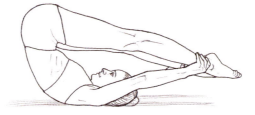

Step 3.

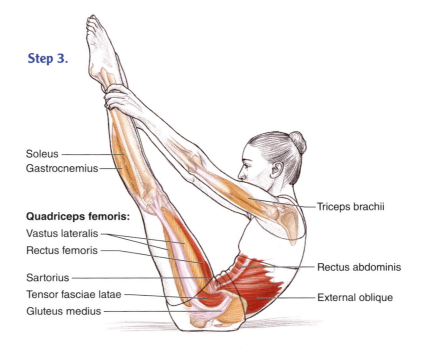

Soleus

Gastrocnemius

Triceps brachii

Quadriceps femoris:

Vastus lateralis

Rectus femoris

Rectus abdominis

Sartorius

Tensor fasciae latae

External oblique

Gluteus medius

Execution

1. *Start position.* Rock back on the sit bones to balance, with the knees close to the chest and open about shoulder-width apart while the lower back is in a C curve. The hands grasp the legs just above the ankles. Straighten both knees to form a V position with the body.
2. *Inhale.* Roll back onto your upper back as shown.
3. *Exhale.* Roll forward to return to the V position. See the main muscle illustration. Repeat the sequence five times.

Targeted Muscles

Spinal flexors and anterior stabilizers: rectus abdominis, external oblique, internal oblique, transversus abdominis

Hip flexors: iliopsoas, rectus femoris, sartorius, tensor fasciae latae, pectineus

Accompanying Muscles

Spinal extensors: erector spinae

Hip extensors: gluteus maximus, hamstrings

Hip abductors: gluteus medius, gluteus minimus

Knee extensors: quadriceps femoris

Ankle–foot plantar flexors: gastrocnemius, soleus

Shoulder flexors: anterior deltoid, pectoralis major (clavicular)

Elbow extensors: triceps brachii

Technique Cues

- In step 1, contract the abdominals to create a slight posterior pelvic tilt and prevent the lower back from arching as the hip flexors contract to help support the legs, especially as the knee extensors straighten the legs. The hip abductors hold the legs apart in the V position while the arms prevent the legs from opening too wide and the shoulder flexors aid the hip flexors in holding the legs off the mat.
- At the beginning of step 2, pull in the lower abdominal wall even farther so that the ASIS rotate posteriorly and the body rolls smoothly onto the upper back.
- As the body rolls back, keep the elbows extended, and use the hip extensors to keep the legs from dropping toward your chest.

(continued)

Rocker With Open Legs (Open-Leg Rocker)   *(continued)*

- At the beginning of step 3, think of using the hip extensors to move your legs away from your chest to help the body roll in the desired direction, although the arms will stop actual change in hip joint angle. As the body rolls forward later in step 3, think of deepening the C curve to assist with rolling as you use the abdominals to pull the front of the rib cage down to help the upper trunk curl up to the balanced V position.

- Throughout the exercise, maintain a long leg line by using the knee extensors to keep the knees straight and the ankle–foot plantar flexors to gently point the feet. Think of reaching your legs out in space.

- Focus on keeping the scapulae in their neutral position. Avoid letting the shoulders rise toward the ears, particularly when in the V position.

- *Imagine.* As suggested by the name of this exercise, imagine the spine is smoothly rocking backward and forward like a rocking chair.

Exercise Notes

Rocker With Open Legs is another signature Pilates exercise, often seen in photos because of its pleasing aesthetics and difficulty. Rocker With Open Legs uses many of the skills practiced in Rolling Back (page 100), but the straight-leg position adds substantial difficulty. This straight-leg position provides a beneficial hamstring stretch for many people and markedly increases the balance challenge. The V position used in this exercise is also an essential element of Teaser (page 92).

Modifications

If your hamstrings are tight, try holding onto the calves rather than the ankles. If this is not enough of an adjustment, allow the knees to bend slightly and hold the backs of the thighs.

Variation

This exercise can also be performed with a flat back as shown. In this variation, pay close attention to extending the spine toward the ceiling on a diagonal while using the abdominals to maintain a neutral pelvic position at the end of the roll-up in step 3. This helps develop the valuable skill of using the spinal extensors to straighten the back without letting the pelvis anteriorly tilt in this demanding position in terms of both balance and leg support.

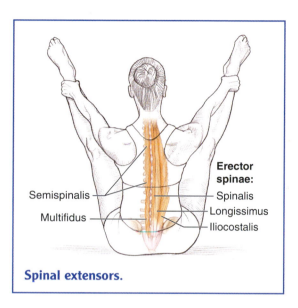

Erector spinae:
Semispinalis
Multifidus
Spinalis
Longissimus
Iliocostalis

Spinal extensors.

Rollover With Legs Spread (Rollover)

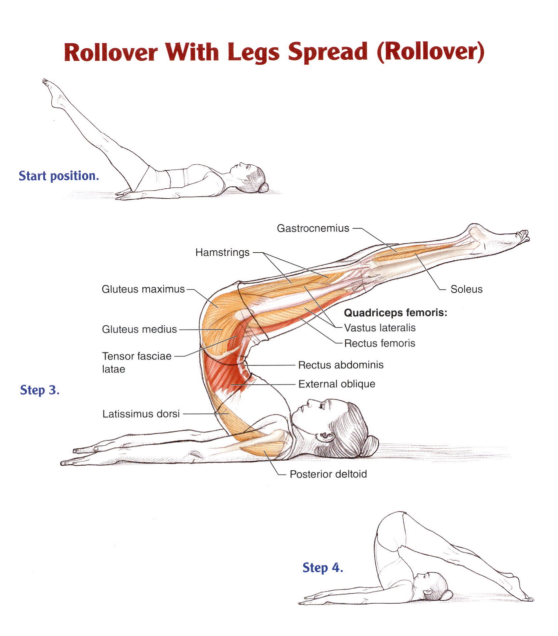

Start position.

Gastrocnemius

Hamstrings

Gluteus maximus

Soleus

Quadriceps femoris:

Gluteus medius

Vastus lateralis

Rectus femoris

Tensor fasciae latae

Rectus abdominis

Step 3.

External oblique

Latissimus dorsi

Posterior deltoid

Step 4.

Execution

1. *Start position.* Lie supine with the arms by the sides and the palms facing down. Hold the legs straight out at an angle of about 60 degrees to the mat or higher if pelvic stability cannot be maintained at 60 degrees.

2. *Inhale.* Raise the legs to a vertical position (90-degree hip flexion).

3. *Exhale.* Round the spine, bringing the pelvis off the mat and toward the shoulders as the legs move over the head as shown in the main muscle illustration.

4. *Inhale.* Lower the feet toward the mat as shown, touching the mat if flexibility allows, and then separate the legs to shoulder-width apart.

5. *Exhale.* Slowly roll the spine back down to the mat. When the pelvis reaches full contact with the mat, lower the legs farther down and bring them back together to return to the start position.

6. Repeat this same sequence, starting with the legs apart in step 1, and then bring them together when overhead in step 4. Roll down with the legs together, and separate them in step 5 as you prepare to repeat the exercise.

7. Repeat the sequence three times starting with the legs together in step 1 and then three times starting with the legs apart.

Targeted Muscles

Spinal flexors: rectus abdominis, external oblique, internal oblique

Hip flexors: iliopsoas, rectus femoris, sartorius, tensor fasciae latae, pectineus

Accompanying Muscles

Anterior spinal stabilizer: transversus abdominis

Hip extensors: gluteus maximus, hamstrings

Hip abductors: gluteus medius, gluteus minimus

Hip adductors: adductor longus, adductor brevis, adductor magnus, gracilis

Knee extensors: quadriceps femoris

Ankle–foot plantar flexors: gastrocnemius, soleus

Shoulder extensors: latissimus dorsi, teres major, posterior deltoid

Technique Cues

- Draw in the abdominal wall toward your spine to help keep the pelvis stable and prevent arching the lower back as the hip flexors hold the legs out and then raise the legs to vertical in steps 1 and 2.

- Use the abdominals to posteriorly tilt the pelvis and round the spine sequentially in early step 3. Start from the bottom of the spine, and maximize lumbar flexion in the rollover phase. People with very flexible spines may need to simultaneously use a subtle contraction of the spinal extensors to achieve the desired C position without the middle and upper back collapsing into too much flexion.

- Use the hip extensors to keep the legs off the mat in step 3 and then to control the legs as they lower to touch the mat in step 4. Use the hip abductors to slightly separate the legs.

(continued)

- Keep the legs close to the chest, and focus on keeping the lower trunk curled as long as possible as the abdominals control the sequential lowering of the spine to the mat in step 5. After the trunk is fully lowered, focus on using the abdominals to keep the pelvis and lower back stable as the hip flexors control the lowering of the legs and the hip adductors bring the legs back together.

- Throughout the exercise, maintain a long leg line by using the knee extensors to keep the knees straight and using the ankle–foot plantar flexors to gently point the feet. Think of reaching the legs out in space in whichever direction the legs are traveling.

- As you raise the pelvis off the mat in step 3, press the arms into the mat to use the shoulder extensors to help bring the upper trunk forward. Pressing the arms into the mat as the trunk lowers to the mat in step 5 will allow the shoulder extensors, working eccentrically, to aid in this challenging phase of the movement.

- *Imagine.* Imagine curling the pelvis around a ball in the up phase of the movement and then scooping the ball toward the feet as the pelvis begins to lower.

Exercise Notes

Think of Rollover With Legs Spread as a reverse movement of Roll-Up (page 73), in which the emphasis is on bringing the pelvis toward the rib cage rather than the rib cage toward the pelvis. Focusing on starting the movement with the pelvis is valuable for developing the skill of spinal articulation in the lower back, with each lumbar vertebra moving sequentially into flexion. It is also useful for developing the skill of using the abdominals to posteriorly tilt the pelvis. This latter skill is essential to counter the tendency of anteriorly tilting the pelvis, a common postural problem that often accompanies movements in which the legs move away from the center, such as in Hundred (page 78) and Teaser (page 92). Posteriorly tilting the pelvis has also been shown to activate more muscle fibers in the lower abdominal area, making such exercises key for developing core stability. Finally, this exercise offers a rigorous dynamic stretch of the hamstrings and spinal extensors for many people.

While Rollover With Legs Spread offers many potential benefits, the motion of bringing the legs over the head can produce weighted flexion of the upper back and neck, which is not appropriate for many people. Be sure to work in a range in which you experience no neck or back discomfort. Consult your physician, and if indicated, delete or modify this exercise as needed.

Modifications

Roll back and lower your legs in steps 3 and 4 only to the point at which you feel the weight of your body primarily supported by the shoulders and upper back, not your neck. This can reduce stress on the neck. If the hamstrings are tight, first work to achieve a position in which your legs are parallel to the mat instead of touching the mat. If hamstring inflexibility prevents this, allow the knees to bend slightly as the legs go overhead. If tightness in the spine or shoulders prevents you from bringing the pelvis above the shoulders in the rollover phase, bend your elbows and use your hands to support your pelvis as the legs reach overhead.

Variation

This exercise can also be performed with the feet flexed (ankle–foot dorsiflexion) in the overhead position to emphasize the dynamic hamstring stretch and the feet pointing as they return to the start position.

Boomerang

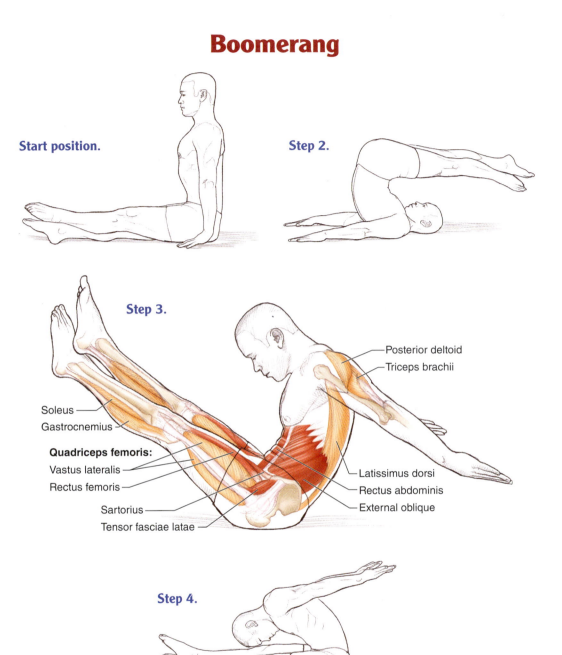

Start position.

Step 2.

Step 3.

Posterior deltoid
Triceps brachii

Soleus
Gastrocnemius

Quadriceps femoris:

Vastus lateralis

Rectus femoris

Sartorius

Tensor fasciae latae

Latissimus dorsi
Rectus abdominis
External oblique

Step 4.

Execution

1. *Start position.* Sit upright with the legs straight to the front, one ankle crossed over the other and the feet pointed. Arms are close to the sides, with palms on the mat.
2. *Exhale.* Roll the torso back onto the mat as shown, legs reaching overhead. See Rollover With Legs Spread (page 112) for key muscles active in the rollover phase. Switch the legs so the opposite ankle is crossed in front.
3. *Inhale.* Roll forward and up into the V position as the arms swing back with the palms facing up. See the main muscle illustration.
4. *Exhale.* Lower the legs to the mat, and bring the head to the knees or as far as flexibility allows as the arms continue to reach back and up as shown.
5. *Inhale.* Maintain this position of the torso as the arms circle around to the front.
6. *Exhale.* Roll back as in step 2. Repeat the sequence six times, alternating the top ankle. After the final repetition, return to start position.

Targeted Muscles

Spinal flexors: rectus abdominis, external oblique, internal oblique

Hip flexors: iliopsoas, rectus femoris, sartorius, tensor fasciae latae, pectineus

Accompanying Muscles

Anterior spinal stabilizer: transversus abdominis

Spinal extensors: erector spinae

Hip extensors: gluteus maximus, hamstrings

Hip abductors: gluteus medius, gluteus minimus

Hip adductors: adductor longus, adductor brevis, adductor magnus, gracilis

Knee extensors: quadriceps femoris

Ankle–foot plantar flexors: gastrocnemius, soleus

Shoulder flexors: anterior deltoid, pectoralis major (clavicular)

Shoulder extensors: latissimus dorsi, teres major, posterior deltoid

Shoulder abductors: middle deltoid, supraspinatus

Elbow extensors: triceps brachii

(continued)

Technique Cues

- Draw the abdominals in and up to prevent arching the lower back as the hip flexors lift the legs off the mat and then to create a posterior pelvic tilt as you roll back in step 2. Think of moving the legs and pelvis together at the beginning of the roll-back. Attempt to keep the angle of hip flexion constant.

- At the end of step 2, use the hip extensors to keep the legs lifted off the mat, and keep the height consistent as they switch. Use the hip abductors to separate the legs slightly and the hip adductors to close them with the new leg in front.

- In step 3, use the abdominals to control the sequential lowering of the pelvis and spine in the first phase and then to help lift the upper trunk into the V position in the later phase. Initially the hip extensors help to bring the legs in the opposite direction, away from the head, before the hip flexors activate to hold the legs off the mat and help raise the trunk into the V position.

- In step 4, use the hip flexors eccentrically to smoothly lower the legs as the abdominals prevent an anterior pelvic tilt. The spinal extensors work eccentrically to control the forward motion (flexion) of the spine.

- Throughout the exercise, maintain a long leg line by using the hip adductors to keep the legs crossed, the knee extensors to keep the knees straight, and the ankle–foot plantar flexors to gently point the feet.

- Press the arms into the mat to encourage use of the shoulder extensors to help raise the upper trunk in step 2 and control its lowering in step 3. In steps 3 and 4, use the shoulder extensors to raise the arms to the back once the arms are no longer in contact with the mat. In these latter steps, think of reaching the arms back and up as they rotate internally to encourage use of the latissimus dorsi while the elbow extensors keep the elbows straight.

- When circling the arms from the back to the front in step 5, the shoulder abductors help the hands clear the mat. Maintain the reach of the arms as they arrive at the front position, using the shoulder flexors eccentrically to lower the arms to the start position.

- *Imagine.* The name of this exercise, Boomerang, provides a useful image for the rhythmic alternating and arc-shaped quality of this movement. After a boomerang flies in an arc in one direction, it reverses direction to arc back to its start point.

Exercise Notes

Boomerang is a complex exercise that dynamically challenges core stability and balance as the whole body moves through space. It involves a large array of muscles but in a manner that promotes whole-body coordination and core control rather than builds strength. It also provides a dynamic stretch for the hamstrings, spinal extensors, and shoulder flexors. Boomerang incorporates the challenges of Rollover With Legs Spread (page 112) and Teaser (page 92) with other elements. Do not attempt this exercise until you achieve proficiency with Rollover With Legs Spread and Teaser. Even then, this is a very advanced exercise and should be performed only if it is appropriate for you.

Modification

If hamstring flexibility is inadequate, slightly bend the knees to relieve the stretch as you roll up to the V position and stretch forward (steps 3 and 4).

Variation

Rather than maintaining a flexed spine, perform this exercise using upper back extension in the V position. Bring the arms forward to an overhead position in step 3, and then circle them to the sides and back. Interlace the hands as shown, and emphasize pulling the shoulder blades slightly down and together as the upper back lifts toward the ceiling. Having the shoulders back instead of rounded forward while reaching the arms back provides a profound stretch for the shoulder flexors. Circle the arms to the sides and forward toward the feet after lowering the legs in step 4.

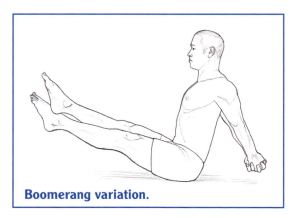

Boomerang variation.

Control Balance

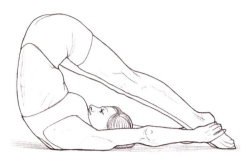

Start position.

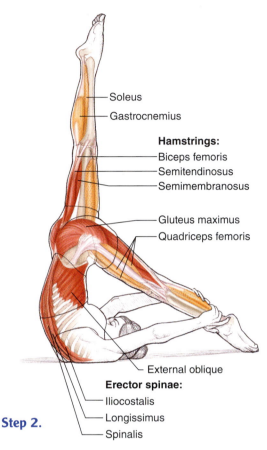

Soleus
Gastrocnemius

Hamstrings:
Biceps femoris
Semitendinosus
Semimembranosus

Gluteus maximus
Quadriceps femoris

External oblique
Erector spinae:
Iliocostalis
Longissimus
Spinalis

Step 2.

Execution

1. *Start position.* Perform Rollover With Legs Spread (page 112), and remain with the legs overhead and the feet gently pointed on the mat or as close to the mat as they can reach. Circle the arms around and overhead to grasp the sides of the feet.

2. *Exhale.* Move the hands so one hand holds the outside ankle of the bottom leg and the other holds the calf. Raise the top leg toward the ceiling, ideally to a vertical position as shown.

3. *Inhale.* Let go of the bottom leg, and switch legs so that the opposite leg reaches toward the ceiling and the hands grasp the outside ankle and calf of the other leg. Repeat the sequence three times on each side, six times in total. After the last repetition, bring both feet to the mat, and roll the spine back down to the mat.

Targeted Muscles

Spinal flexors: rectus abdominis, external oblique, internal oblique

Spinal extensors: erector spinae (spinalis, longissimus, iliocostalis), semispinalis, deep posterior spinal group

Hip extensors: gluteus maximus, hamstrings (semimembranosus, semitendinosus, biceps femoris)

Accompanying Muscles

Anterior spinal stabilizer: transversus abdominis

Hip flexors: iliopsoas, rectus femoris

Knee extensors: quadriceps femoris

Ankle–foot plantar flexors: gastrocnemius, soleus

Shoulder flexors: anterior deltoid, pectoralis major (clavicular)

Technique Cues

- When the legs are overhead in step 1, focus on using the abdominals to maintain a C curve of the spine and keep the pelvis over the shoulders. Simultaneously, use a small contraction of the very low spinal extensors to decrease the posterior tilt of the pelvis, and think of reaching the coccyx toward the ceiling. Try to keep this core positioning stable as the legs alternately lift and lower.

- As one leg reaches toward the ceiling in step 2, focus on using the hip extensors to raise the back of the thigh to be in line with the pelvis. As the legs switch in step 3, smoothly control the lowering of the top leg with an eccentric contraction of the hip extensors, while the same muscle group in the other leg is used concentrically to raise the leg.

- To aid with stability, use the shoulder flexors to pull down on the ankle of the lower leg. By keeping the lower leg stable, the hip flexors also can be used to prevent the trunk from falling back down toward the mat.

- Throughout the exercise, maintain a long leg line by using the knee extensors to keep the knees straight and the ankle–foot plantar flexors to gently point the feet.

- *Imagine.* Imagine the legs are like a protractor. The lower leg is the arm of the protractor that remains stationary. The upper leg is the arm of the protractor that moves to a vertical position.

(continued)

Control Balance   *(continued)*

Exercise Notes

Control Balance is a very challenging exercise that develops control of the core to maintain balance, even though reaching one leg to the ceiling will tend to make the trunk want to fall back toward the mat. An intricate activation of the abdominals, spinal extensors, hip extensors, and hip flexors is required to execute this exercise without losing balance. In addition, the leg movement offers potential benefits in terms of dynamic flexibility for the often tight hamstrings and hip flexors.

While offering strong potential benefits, this exercise intensifies the risks of imposing weighted flexion on the upper back and neck mentioned in Rollover With Legs Spread (page 112) and is better avoided until you receive medical clearance that it is appropriate for you.

Modification

If flexibility in the hamstrings is slightly insufficient to achieve step 2, hold the lower leg stationary with the foot above, not touching, the mat. If hamstring and lower back tightness is extreme, first develop adequate flexibility with other Pilates exercises such as Rollover With Legs Spread (page 112).

Variation

Perform the exercise with the foot on the mat flexed (ankle–foot dorsiflexion) and a gentle double pulse and associated two percussive exhales (as used with Single Straight-Leg Stretch, page 84) when the top leg is at its peak height, while using the inhale for the leg switch.

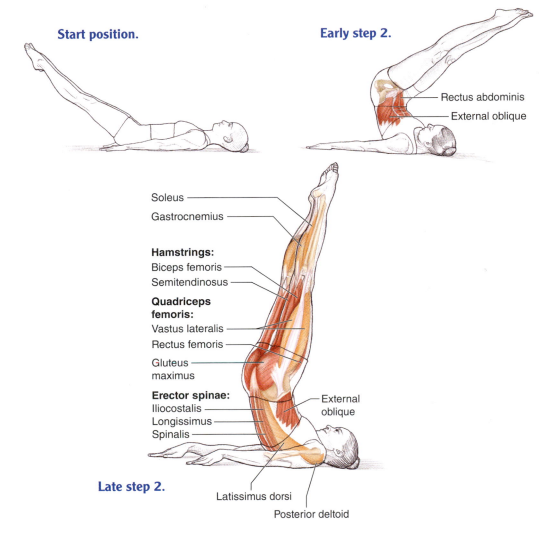

Jackknife

Start position.

Early step 2.

Rectus abdominis

External oblique

Soleus

Gastrocnemius

Hamstrings:
Biceps femoris
Semitendinosus

Quadriceps femoris:
Vastus lateralis
Rectus femoris

Gluteus maximus

Erector spinae:
Iliocostalis
Longissimus
Spinalis

External oblique

Late step 2.

Latissimus dorsi

Posterior deltoid

Execution

1. *Start position.* Lie supine with the arms by the sides and the palms facing down. Hold the legs straight out at an angle of about 60 degrees relative to the mat or higher if pelvic stability cannot be maintained at 60 degrees. Gently point the feet. From this position, raise the legs to vertical (90-degree hip flexion).

2. *Inhale.* Round the spine and bring the pelvis and lower back off the mat, with the legs on a diagonal line opposite your face as shown in the first muscle illustration. Lift the legs and pelvis toward the ceiling as shown in the second muscle illustration.

3. *Exhale.* Slowly roll the trunk down to the mat. When the pelvis comes in full contact with the mat, bring the legs back to the vertical start position. Repeat the sequence five times.

(continued)

Targeted Muscles

Spinal flexors: rectus abdominis, external oblique, internal oblique

Spinal extensors: erector spinae (spinalis, longissimus, iliocostalis), semi-spinalis, deep posterior spinal group

Hip flexors: iliopsoas, rectus femoris, sartorius, tensor fasciae latae, pectineus

Hip extensors: gluteus maximus, hamstrings (semimembranosus, semitendinosus, biceps femoris)

Accompanying Muscles

Anterior spinal stabilizer: transversus abdominis

Hip adductors: adductor longus, adductor brevis, adductor magnus, gracilis

Knee extensors: quadriceps femoris

Ankle–foot plantar flexors: gastrocnemius, soleus

Shoulder extensors: latissimus dorsi, teres major, posterior deltoid

Technique Cues

- Draw the abdominal wall in toward your spine to help keep the pelvis stable and prevent undesired arching of the lower back as the hip flexors hold the legs out and then raise the legs to vertical in step 1.
- Early in step 2, use the abdominals to posteriorly tilt the pelvis and curl the spine sequentially off the mat, starting from the bottom. Also use the hip extensors to keep the legs on a diagonal instead of allowing them to drop to the mat and then to raise the legs toward the ceiling late in step 2.
- As the legs rise, simultaneously press the arms into the mat to use the shoulder extensors to bring the upper trunk forward while the spinal extensors help lengthen the back toward the ceiling so the feet are over the face but most of the body weight is supported by the shoulders.
- Control the body as it lowers back to the start position in step 3. Focus on using the abdominals to control the release of the posterior tilt to a neutral position toward the end of the movement.
- Throughout the movement, think of gently pulling the inner thighs together to activate the hip adductors, as the knee extensors keep the knees straight and the ankle–foot plantar flexors point the feet to achieve a long, arrowlike leg line.
- *Imagine.* As the name implies, the image of opening and closing a jackknife can be helpful in achieving the desired precise opening (extension) and closing (flexion) at the hip joint.

Exercise Notes

Jackknife shares many of the benefits of Rollover With Legs Spread (page 112), such as a dynamic stretch for the hamstrings and lower spinal extensors. But it offers a greater spinal articulation challenge by incorporating extension of the spine between phases of flexion and greater balance skill when both legs are lifted to the ceiling. This use of spinal extension is helpful for spinal muscle balance and is a valuable respite for the many other Pilates exercises that focus on spinal flexion alone.

Modification

Use the arms to support the pelvis as shown, and bring the feet overhead only as far as lower back and hamstring flexibility allow. This modification reduces the weight borne by the neck. However, check with your doctor to see if this exercise or its modification is appropriate for you.

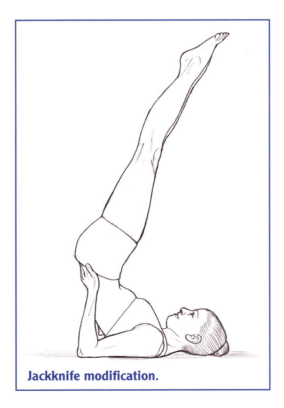

Jackknife modification.

Variation

After you develop proficiency, and only if it is appropriate for your body, try lowering the feet to touch the mat in step 2 and raising the trunk to a more vertical position as you lift the legs toward the ceiling.

BRIDGING FOR
A FUNCTIONAL SPINE

Research has demonstrated that drawing the abdominal wall inward tends to produce activation of the transversus abdominis and internal oblique muscles. As discussed in chapter 2, these muscles have been shown to be very important for core stability and protection of the lower back. Hence, pulling in the abdominal wall, hollowing, and scooping (typically accompanying spinal flexion) are commonly used as cues in Pilates exercises to develop desired activation of these key muscles.

However, many functional movements used in everyday life do not involve or permit a scooping inward motion of the abdominal wall, yet core stability is still vital. Therefore, this chapter includes exercises that focus on keeping the pelvis and spine stable while the spine is neutral or slightly arched (spinal hyperextension) rather than scooped (spinal flexion). This demands a subtle, coordinated contraction of both the abdominals and spinal extensors, sometimes termed *bracing*. Some researchers hold that training to incorporate bracing is essential for protecting the spine during lifting, athletics, and other activities that involve large forces.

The exercises in this chapter also share the characteristic that the pelvis is not resting on the mat but rather is lifted off the mat so the trunk forms a bridge shape, with the limbs helping to provide support structures for this bridge. In rehabilitation, the term *bridging* often refers to exercises in which the hip extensors, particularly the hamstrings and gluteus maximus, are used to lift the pelvis from the mat. The hip extensors are very important for posterior stability of the pelvis, and Shoulder Bridge (page 128) and Leg Pull (page 138) fit this more traditional description of bridging. However, these two exercises differ from each other in that Leg Pull uses a neutral position of the spine and pelvis while Shoulder Bridge uses a slightly arched position of the spine. In addition, the arms are bent as they support the trunk in Shoulder Bridge. This arched position of the spine and use of arm support is shared by two other exercises, Scissors (page 131) and Bicycle (page 134). However, in Shoulder Bridge one leg also helps support, while in Scissors and Bicycle both legs are in the air, moving with a split action or cycling action. The hands provide crucial support for the pelvis throughout. All of these exercises share the key challenge of maintaining stability of the spine and pelvis, with the spine in a neutral or slightly arched position while one or both legs move through space.

The last two exercises of this chapter, Leg Pull Front (page 142) and Push-Up (page 145), share the characteristic of the pelvis being lifted off the mat, with the limbs acting as support structures. However, they differ from the earlier exercises in this chapter in that the trunk is facing down versus up. In this position, gravity tends to make the lower back arch and the hips extend. Therefore, a slightly different use of core muscles is required to keep the pelvis and spine neutral and stable as one leg lifts and lowers in Leg Pull Front or the arms bend and straighten in Push-Up.

Shoulder Bridge

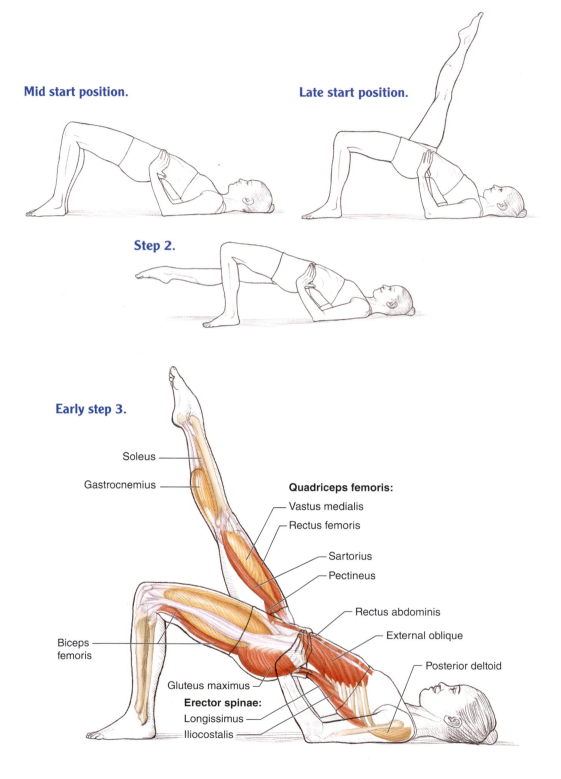

Mid start position.

Late start position.

Step 2.

Early step 3.

Soleus

Gastrocnemius

Quadriceps femoris:

Vastus medialis

Rectus femoris

Sartorius

Pectineus

Rectus abdominis

External oblique

Posterior deltoid

Biceps femoris

Gluteus maximus

Erector spinae:

Longissimus

Iliocostalis

Execution

1. *Start position.* Lie supine with the knees bent and the feet flat on the mat, hip-width apart. Place the arms by the sides with the palms facing down. Curl the pelvis off the mat, and place the palm of each hand at the waist, fingers facing inward, with the hands helping to support the weight of the trunk as shown. Lift one foot off the mat, bringing the knee toward the chest, and then straighten the knee so that the leg is reaching toward the ceiling with the foot gently pointed as shown.

2. *Exhale.* Lower the up-stretched leg down toward the mat as shown.

3. *Inhale.* Lift the leg back up (as shown in the main muscle illustration), ending in a vertical position. Repeat the sequence five times. Return to the mid start position. Perform the same sequence five times on the opposite leg. Finish by rolling the pelvis down to the initial start position.

Targeted Muscles

Posterior spinal stabilizers: erector spinae (spinalis, longissimus, iliocostalis), semispinalis, deep posterior spinal group

Anterior spinal stabilizers: rectus abdominis, external oblique, internal oblique, transversus abdominis

Hip extensors: gluteus maximus, hamstrings (semimembranosus, semitendinosus, biceps femoris)

Hip flexors: iliopsoas, rectus femoris, sartorius, tensor fascia latae, pectineus

Accompanying Muscles

Knee extensors: quadriceps femoris

Ankle–foot plantar flexors: gastrocnemius, soleus

Shoulder extensors: latissimus dorsi, teres major, posterior deltoid

Scapular adductors: trapezius, rhomboids

Technique Cues

- In the start position, press the feet into the mat and think of lifting the bottom of the pelvis toward the ceiling to emphasize use of the hip extensors, especially the hamstrings, as previously discussed with Pelvic Curl (page 52). The knee extensors also help raise the thighs. Then use the hip flexors followed by the knee extensors to bring one leg to a vertical position.

- Focus on pressing the upper arms down into the mat and lifting the chest to encourage use of the shoulder extensors and spinal extensors. This will aid with arching the back and lifting the pelvis high enough to allow the hands to provide support.

(continued)

Shoulder Bridge   *(continued)*

- Simultaneously, focus on pulling the lower attachment of the abdominals up to prevent the pelvis from tilting forward too far and to help maintain stability of the spine and pelvis throughout the exercise.
- While core stability is maintained, think of keeping the moving leg long. Use the knee extensors to maintain a straight knee and the ankle–foot plantar flexors to keep the foot pointed. At the same time, use the hip extensors in step 2 to initiate lowering the leg, followed rapidly by using the hip flexors to control the continued lowering of the leg. The hip flexors then begin to raise the leg back up in step 3.
- *Imagine.* Imagine your spine is arching like a Japanese bridge over a river while one leg moves without disrupting this stable, strong arch.

Exercise Notes

This exercise offers an advanced challenge to pelvic stability since the pelvis is off the mat as one leg supports the body and the other leg moves up and down through a large range of motion. In addition, the spine is arched slightly, so extra care must be taken to keep the pelvis stationary as the leg lowers, further described in Scissors (page 131). If adequate stability is maintained, this exercise also offers dynamic flexibility benefits for the hamstring and hip flexor muscles.

Modification

If you are unable to maintain pelvic stability, try performing the exercise with the pelvis slightly tilted posteriorly as described in the variation, and move the leg through a smaller range.

Variation

You can perform this exercise with the pelvis raised off the mat with a slight posterior pelvic tilt and without hand support. The foot can be flexed as the leg rises (ankle–foot dorsiflexion) to emphasize a dynamic hamstring stretch at the top of the movement.

Scissors

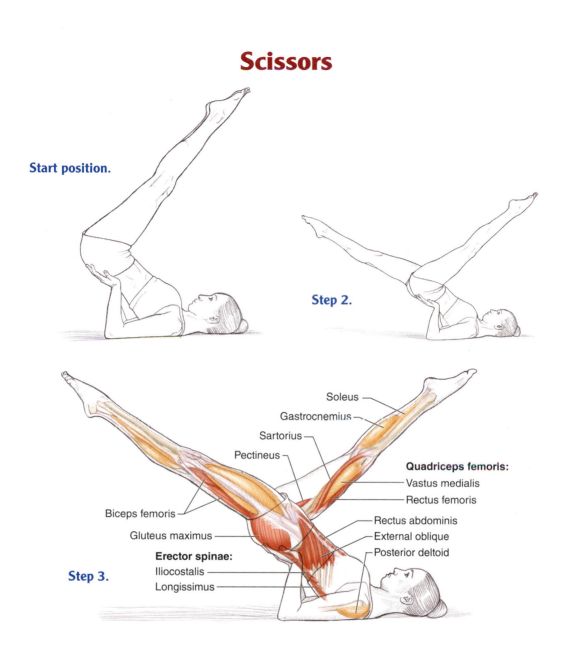

Start position.

Step 2.

Step 3.

Soleus

Gastrocnemius

Sartorius

Pectineus

Quadriceps femoris:

Vastus medialis

Rectus femoris

Biceps femoris

Gluteus maximus

Rectus abdominis

External oblique

Posterior deltoid

Erector spinae:

Iliocostalis

Longissimus

Execution

1. *Start position.* Lie supine with the arms by the sides and the palms facing down. The legs are held straight out at an angle of about 60 degrees relative to the mat or higher if pelvic stability cannot be maintained at 60 degrees. Raise the legs and curl the pelvis off the mat until the feet are above the head. Place the heel of each hand toward the back of the waistline, with the fingers pointing down toward the coccyx. Allow the pelvis to lower slightly so the hands help support the weight of the pelvis while the lower back is slightly arched (spinal hyperextension).

2. *Inhale.* Lower one leg while the other leg continues to reach overhead to form a split position as shown.

(continued)

3. *Exhale.* Switch the legs as shown in the main muscle illustration. Repeat the sequence 5 times on each leg, 10 times in total. Finish by bringing the legs together as in the start position and rolling down to the mat.

Targeted Muscles

Posterior spinal stabilizers: erector spinae (spinalis, longissimus, iliocostalis), semispinalis, deep posterior spinal group

Anterior spinal stabilizers: rectus abdominis, external oblique, internal oblique, transversus abdominis

Hip flexors: iliopsoas, rectus femoris, sartorius, tensor fasciae latae, pectineus

Hip extensors: gluteus maximus, hamstrings (semimembranosus, semitendinosus, biceps femoris)

Accompanying Muscles

Knee extensors: quadriceps femoris

Ankle–foot plantar flexors: gastrocnemius, soleus

Shoulder extensors: latissimus dorsi, teres major, posterior deltoid

Scapular adductors: trapezius, rhomboids

Technique Cues

- In step 1, think of pulling up the front and back of the pelvis simultaneously so that the posterior spinal stabilizers and abdominals cocontract appropriately to create a slight arch of the lower back. Maintain this position of the spine and a stable pelvis throughout the exercise.

- Concentrate on using the scapular adductors to pull the scapulae together slightly rather than letting the shoulders round forward. Continue pressing the arms down into the mat to encourage use of the shoulder extensors to help keep the upper trunk lifted off the mat.

- Reach your legs in opposite directions in steps 2 and 3 while maintaining a completely still trunk. Use the knee extensors to keep the knees straight and the ankle–foot plantar flexors to keep the feet pointed to help achieve the desired long leg line.

- To initiate the switch from step 2 to step 3, raise the bottom leg with the hip flexors and initiate the lowering of the top leg with the hip extensors. After the legs pass vertical, the opposite muscles then become important for controlling the legs as they work against gravity.

- At the end of the split, emphasize the opposition of using the hip flexors to reach up with the top leg while using the hip extensors to reach down with the bottom leg. This opposition can help maintain core stability while maximizing the range of the legs to achieve the desired stretch of the hamstrings of the top leg and the hip flexors of the bottom leg simultaneously.

ADVANCED

- *Imagine.* As the name of the exercise suggests, the switching of the legs should have a brisk dynamic, like opening and closing scissors, with the motion isolated to the hips.

Exercise Notes

This exercise offers many similar benefits to Shoulder Bridge (page 128), with a greater challenge to pelvic stability because both legs are off the mat and moving through a large range of motion. As with Shoulder Bridge, the pelvis is held off the mat with arm support while the back is slightly arched. Therefore, skilled stabilization of the spine and pelvis is essential for protecting the lower back and reaping the potential dynamic flexibility benefits for the hamstrings and hip flexors.

Hip flexor stretch. As described in Leg Lift Supine (page 56), the hip flexors, including the strong iliopsoas, have attachments onto the front of the pelvis and the spine. When the leg lowers and the resting length of the iliopsoas is approached, the stretch applied to the muscle can easily pull the pelvis forward, while the iliopsoas remains at approximately the same length. However, if the pelvis is held stationary, further lowering of the leg will lengthen the muscle (i.e.,

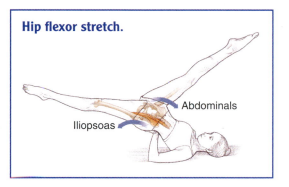

Hip flexor stretch.

Abdominals

Iliopsoas

create a dynamic stretch). Learning to stabilize the pelvis so that an effective stretch can be applied to the iliopsoas is an important skill since tight hip flexors are associated with postural problems such as an arched lower back (lumbar hyperlordosis). Furthermore, many Pilates exercises such as Hundred (page 78) and Rollover With Legs Spread (page 112) use the hip flexors to support the legs off the mat in a relatively small range of movement, potentially resulting in tightness of the hip flexors. Therefore, exercises that incorporate a dynamic stretch are valuable for helping to prevent tightness of these key postural muscles.

Modification

If you are unable to maintain pelvic stability or if you experience any back discomfort, try performing the exercise with the pelvis and lower back in a neutral position and the hands positioned above the pelvis to support the lower back.

Variation

Following Rollover With Legs Spread (page 112) in step 1, bend the knees to create a ball shape with the body. Place the hands under the pelvis for support, and then straighten the legs to a vertical position. Stretch the legs in opposite directions, performing a double pulse in the split position accompanied by an exhale, while the leg switch occurs on the inhale. This is similar to the pattern used in Single Straight-Leg Stretch (page 84). In the split position, each leg should be equidistant from the vertical line, creating an even V shape.

Bicycle

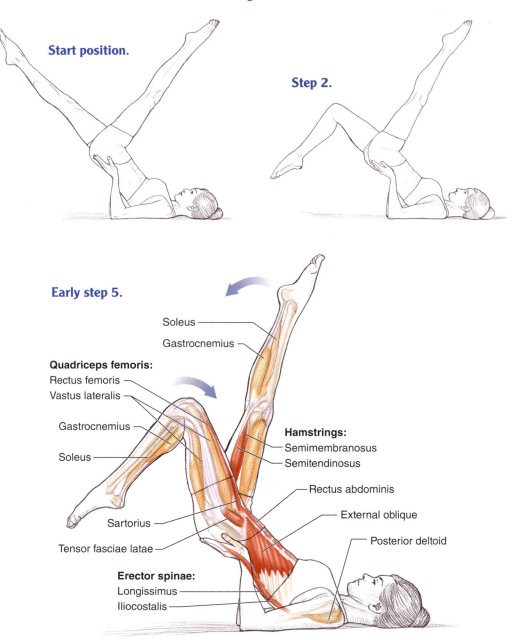

Start position.

Step 2.

Early step 5.

Soleus

Gastrocnemius

Quadriceps femoris:
Rectus femoris
Vastus lateralis

Gastrocnemius

Soleus

Sartorius

Tensor fasciae latae

Erector spinae:
Longissimus
Iliocostalis

Hamstrings:
Semimembranosus
Semitendinosus

Rectus abdominis

External oblique

Posterior deltoid

Execution

1. *Start position.* Start in the same position as for Scissors (page 131), with the legs in the split position as shown.
2. *Inhale.* Bend the bottom leg, bringing the heel toward the buttocks as shown.
3. *Exhale.* Raise the bottom leg toward your chest with the knee bent while the top leg lowers with the knee straight. Then straighten the top leg to create the split position.
4. *Inhale.* Bend the bottom leg, bringing the heel toward the buttocks while the top leg reaches overhead.
5. *Exhale.* Raise the bottom leg toward your chest with the knee bent while lowering the top leg with the knee straight. See the main muscle illustration. Then straighten the top leg to create the split position. Repeat the sequence 5 times on each leg, 10 times in total.

Targeted Muscles

Posterior spinal stabilizers: erector spinae (spinalis, longissimus, iliocostalis), semispinalis, deep posterior spinal group

Anterior spinal stabilizers: rectus abdominis, external oblique, internal oblique, transversus abdominis

Hip flexors: iliopsoas, rectus femoris, sartorius, tensor fasciae latae, pectineus

Hip extensors: gluteus maximus, hamstrings (semimembranosus, semitendinosus, biceps femoris)

Accompanying Muscles

Knee flexors: hamstrings

Knee extensors: quadriceps femoris

Ankle–foot plantar flexors: gastrocnemius, soleus

Shoulder extensors: latissimus dorsi, teres major, posterior deltoid

Scapular adductors: trapezius, rhomboids

Technique Cues

- As with Scissors (page 131), in step 1 think of pulling up the front and back of the pelvis simultaneously so that the abdominals and posterior spinal stabilizers work together to create a slight arch of the lower back. Maintain this position of the spine and a stable pelvis throughout the exercise.
- Concentrate on using the scapular adductors to pull the scapulae slightly together rather than letting the shoulders round forward. Also focus on pressing the elbows down into the mat to encourage use of the shoulder extensors to keep the upper trunk lifted off the mat.

(continued)

Bicycle   *(continued)*

- While maintaining a stable trunk, reach both legs out in opposite directions in the split position. Use the knee extensors to straighten the knees and the ankle–foot plantar flexors to point the feet to help achieve the desired long leg line.

- In steps 2 and 4, the hip extensors keep the bottom leg close to the mat while the hamstrings also function as knee flexors to bend the knee. Simultaneously, think of continuing to reach the top leg above the head to encourage adequate use of the hip flexors, similar to Scissors (page 131). This also will help prevent the movements of the bottom leg from pulling down the top leg.

- In steps 3 and 5, think of drawing the bottom knee up toward your chest, initially using the hip flexors. At the same time, reach the top leg over and down, initially using the hip extensors. As the legs cross vertical, the opposite muscles will be used to control the legs as they work against gravity. Use the knee extensors to straighten the top leg. At the end of this phase, the muscles that initiated the movement will be used again to achieve a maximum split position and apply the desired stretch to the hamstrings of the top leg and hip flexors of the bottom leg.

- *Imagine.* As the name of the exercise suggests, the movement of the legs should be smooth, rhythmic, and coordinated, like cycling on a bicycle with very large pedals and wheels.

Exercise Notes

This exercise builds on the challenge of Scissors (page 131) by adding complexity to the leg movement. This makes it more difficult to maintain stability of the pelvis and lower back in the arched position. Similar to Scissors, when properly performed, Bicycle also offers dynamic flexibility benefits for the hip flexors and hamstrings.

Modification

If you are unable to maintain pelvic stability or if you experience any back discomfort, try performing the exercise with the pelvis and lower back in a neutral position and the hands positioned above the pelvis to support the lower back.

Variation

This exercise can also be performed with greater lumbar hyperextension as shown. In this variation, the goal is to touch the mat with the toes of the bottom leg as the knee bends while maintaining core stability. This variation is good preparation for many more advanced Pilates exercises that focus on using the spinal extensors with cocontraction of the abdominals, such as Rocking (page 187) and Swan Dive (page 190). However, this variation should not be performed if you experience back discomfort or if you have a back condition and have been told by your physician to avoid spinal hyperextension.

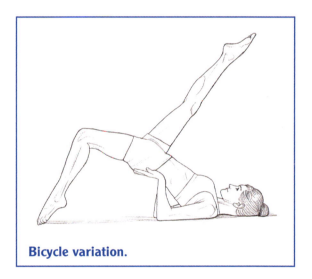

Bicycle variation.

Leg Pull

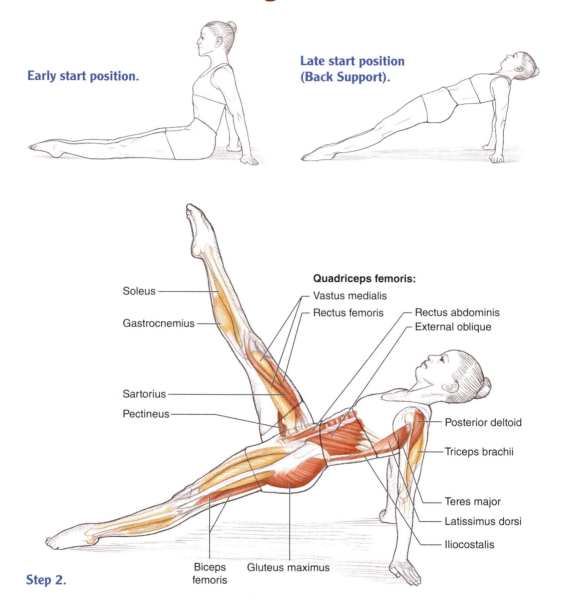

Early start position.

**Late start position
(Back Support).**

Soleus

Gastrocnemius

Sartorius

Pectineus

Quadriceps femoris:

Vastus medialis

Rectus femoris

Rectus abdominis

External oblique

Posterior deltoid

Triceps brachii

Teres major

Latissimus dorsi

Iliocostalis

Biceps
femoris

Gluteus maximus

Step 2.

Execution

1. *Start position.* Sit with the legs together and outstretched to the front, with the feet pointed as shown. The arms are straight and behind the trunk, fingers pointing sideways. Lift the pelvis off the mat to form a straight line from the sides of the ankles through the knees, hips, and shoulders as shown. This position is sometimes called Back Support.
2. *Inhale.* Raise one leg toward the ceiling.
3. *Exhale.* Lower that leg back to the mat.
4. *Inhale.* Raise the other leg toward the ceiling.
5. *Exhale.* Lower that leg back to the mat. Repeat the sequence 5 times on each leg, 10 times in total.

Targeted Muscles

Posterior spinal stabilizers: erector spinae (spinalis, longissimus, iliocostalis), semispinalis, deep posterior spinal group

Anterior spinal stabilizers: rectus abdominis, external oblique, internal oblique, transversus abdominis

Hip extensors: gluteus maximus, hamstrings (semimembranosus, semitendinosus, biceps femoris)

Hip flexors: iliopsoas, rectus femoris, sartorius, tensor fasciae latae, pectineus

Shoulder extensors: latissimus dorsi, teres major, posterior deltoid

Scapular depressors: lower trapezius, serratus anterior

Scapular adductors: trapezius, rhomboids, levator scapulae

Accompanying Muscles

Knee extensors: quadriceps femoris

Ankle–foot plantar flexors: gastrocnemius, soleus

Elbow extensors: triceps brachii

Technique Cues

- In step 1, focus on pressing the feet into the mat and lifting the bottom of the pelvis toward the ceiling to emphasize use of the hip extensors, particularly the hamstrings. This will help achieve the desired straight-line position. Simultaneously, press the hands down into the mat to encourage use of the shoulder extensors to aid in lifting the upper trunk. The anterior and posterior spinal stabilizers should maintain a neutral pelvis and spine.
- As one leg is raised in steps 2 and 4 and lowered in steps 3 and 5, primarily through concentric and then eccentric action of the hip flexors, emphasize keeping the opposite side of the pelvis lifted, stationary, and neutral.

(continued)

Leg Pull   *(continued)*

- Throughout the exercise, maintain a long line with both legs, using the knee extensors to keep the knees straight and the ankle–foot plantar flexors to keep the feet pointed. Be careful to avoid hyperextending the knee of the support leg.

- While the arms press down to emphasize continuous use of the shoulder extensors, also focus on keeping the elbows straight through use of the elbow extensors. However, avoid hyperextending the elbows. Simultaneously, emphasize keeping the scapulae down through use of the scapular depressors, and the shoulder blades back through use of the scapular adductors.

- *Imagine.* To help achieve the desired stability, imagine that your trunk, arms, and support leg form a bridge, and guy wires of the bridge pull the bottom of the pelvis upward so that a solid form is maintained as the moving leg swings freely up and down.

Exercise Notes

Leg Pull shares many of the benefits of Shoulder Bridge (page 128), including a dynamic hamstring stretch, but it uses a neutral position of the pelvis and spine rather than a slightly arched position. Leg Pull also requires that the pelvis remain lifted off the mat without support from the hands and that the body be supported with the arms and legs straight. This is more challenging for trunk stabilization. The longer lever created by the support leg requires that the hip extensors work harder to keep the pelvis lifted, and it offers valuable additional potential strength and endurance benefits for the hip extensors. The straight position of the arms also requires greater shoulder range of motion, providing a valuable stretch for the shoulder flexors for many people. However, supporting the body with straight limbs requires that you pay more attention to good form. Avoid knee or elbow hyperextension and excessive elevation of the scapulae or rounding forward of the shoulders. It may be helpful to use the preparatory exercise described in the modification section.

Scapular depression. As the trunk is lifted to the straight-line position, the shoulders move into extreme extension. Shoulder extension is linked naturally with elevation of the scapulae, so it is easy to allow the shoulders to lift toward the ears. Use the scapular depressors, particularly the lower trapezius and lower fibers of the serratus anterior (see the illustration), to minimize this elevation. The trapezius is on the back of the body, and its contraction alone tends to pinch the scapulae together (scapular adduction, or retraction). The serratus anterior's forward attachments are on the sides of the rib cage, and its contraction alone tends to pull the scapulae toward the sides and front of the body (scapular abduction, or protraction). But coordinated contraction of these muscles will allow the desired scapular depression, with the scapulae also remaining the appropriate neutral distance from the spine rather than separating with the shoulders rolling forward. In step 1, focus on pulling the scapulae down slightly before lifting the trunk to help activate these muscles. Coordinated use of the trapezius and serratus anterior plays a key role in optimal use of the arms in many Pilates exercises.

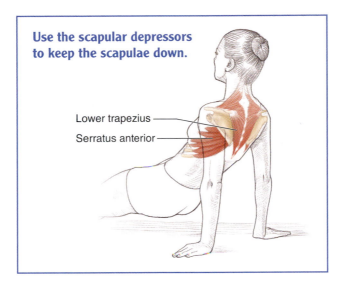

Use the scapular depressors to keep the scapulae down.

Lower trapezius

Serratus anterior

Modification

Perform only step 1 (Back Support), repeatedly lifting the body from sitting to the straight-line position and lowering the pelvis back to the mat with good control and form. After developing proficiency, add raising and lowering one leg, which is Leg Pull. Back Support can be used as a warm-up before execution of Leg Pull or as an exercise in itself.

Variations

This exercise can also be performed with the arms rotated inward so that the fingers point toward the pelvis. This position can be useful to prepare for more advanced exercises done on the Pilates apparatus. In addition, you can perform consecutive repetitions of raising and lowering the leg on the same side before switching sides. Consecutive repetitions can provide greater muscular strength and endurance benefits for the hip extensors.

Leg Pull Front

**Start position
(Front Support).**

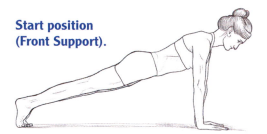

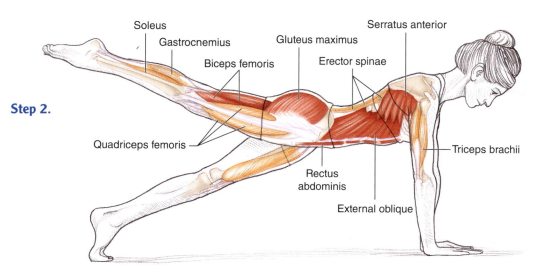

Step 2.

Soleus

Gastrocnemius

Biceps femoris

Gluteus maximus

Serratus anterior

Erector spinae

Quadriceps femoris

Rectus
abdominis

External oblique

Triceps brachii

Execution

1. *Start position.* Start with the body weight supported on the hands and toes, knees and elbows straight. The hands are directly under the shoulders, with the fingers pointing forward. The body is in plank position so the sides of the ankles, knees, pelvis, shoulders, and ears are approximately in a straight line. (This is commonly called Front Support.)

2. *Inhale.* Raise one leg toward the ceiling. See the main muscle illustration.

3. *Exhale.* Lower that leg back to the mat.

4. *Inhale.* Raise the opposite leg toward the ceiling.

5. *Exhale.* Lower that leg back to the mat. Repeat the sequence 5 times on each leg, 10 times in total.

Targeted Muscles

Anterior spinal stabilizers: rectus abdominis, external oblique, internal oblique, transversus abdominis

Hip extensors: gluteus maximus, hamstrings (semimembranosus, semitendinosus, biceps femoris)

Scapular abductors: serratus anterior, pectoralis minor

Accompanying Muscles

Posterior spinal stabilizers: erector spinae

Knee extensors: quadriceps femoris

Ankle–foot plantar flexors: gastrocnemius, soleus

Ankle–foot dorsiflexors: tibialis anterior, extensor digitorum longus

Shoulder flexors: anterior deltoid, pectoralis major (clavicular)

Elbow extensors: triceps brachii

Technique Cues

- Throughout the exercise, focus on pressing into the mat with the arms while the elbow extensors keep the elbows straight. This focus encourages use of the scapular abductors to keep the scapulae wide and the shoulder flexors to keep the chest lifted above the arms. Concentrate on using the abdominals to stabilize the lower back and pelvis.

- In steps 2 and 4, reach the leg out while using the hip extensors to lift the leg, the knee extensors to keep the knee straight, and the ankle–foot plantar flexors to point the foot. Focus on keeping the pelvis facing the mat through use of the obliques so that the lift of the leg does not rotate the pelvis. Also, use the abdominals to allow only a slight anterior tilt of the pelvis as the leg reaches its high point to the back.

- In steps 3 and 5, return the pelvis to a neutral position as primarily the hip extensors act eccentrically to control lowering the leg and the ankle–foot dorsiflexors flex the foot as it returns to the mat.

- *Imagine.* Imagine that the arms, trunk, and support leg form a sturdy bridge that remains solid as the other leg lifts and lowers.

(continued)

Leg Pull Front   *(continued)*

Exercise Notes

This exercise offers a different challenge to pelvic stability than do prior exercises in this chapter in that the trunk is turned toward the mat rather than toward the ceiling. The desired neutral starting position requires skilled activation of the abdominals to counter the tendency of gravity to make the lower back arch and the pelvis anteriorly tilt; excessive activation of the abdominals would produce undesired rounding (flexion) of the spine. Lifting one leg can provide some toning benefits for the hip extensors as well as produce a greater stability challenge. If adequate pelvic stability is maintained, this exercise offers dynamic flexibility benefits for the hip flexors as described in Scissors (page 131). Furthermore, Leg Pull Front offers a valuable opportunity to develop vital scapular stabilization needed for any positions involving front support or pushing-type movements as well as for prevention of the postural condition termed *winged scapulae*.

Stabilization with the scapular abductors. In Front Support described in step 1, gravity tends to make the scapulae pinch close together toward the spine (scapular adduction, or retraction). The scapular abductors, particularly the serratus anterior, must counter this effect and maintain the desired wide, neutral position of the scapulae. Failure to stabilize the scapulae will markedly diminish the potential value of this exercise.

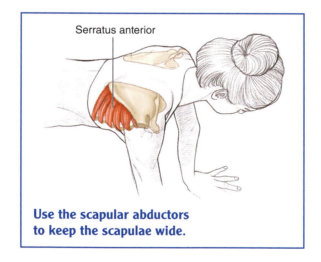

Serratus anterior

Use the scapular abductors to keep the scapulae wide.

Push-Up

Early start position.

Mid start position.

Late start position (Front Support).

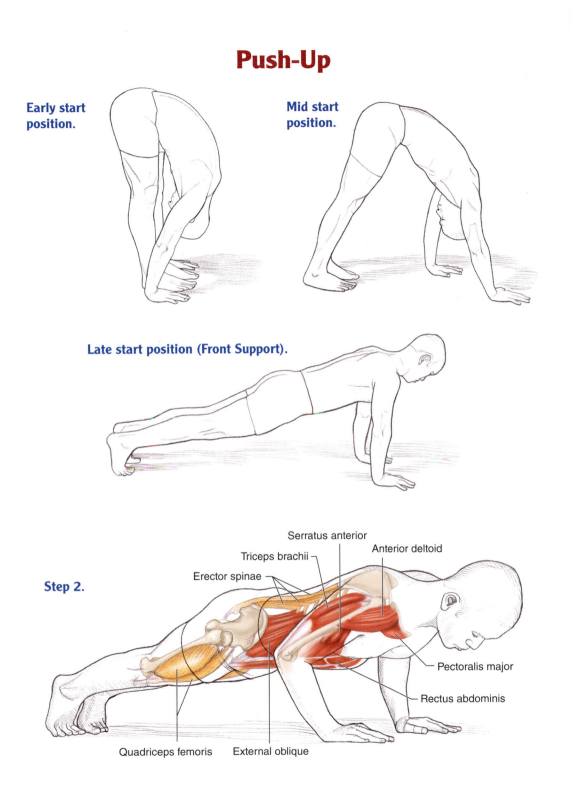

Step 2.

Serratus anterior

Triceps brachii

Anterior deltoid

Erector spinae

Pectoralis major

Rectus abdominis

Quadriceps femoris

External oblique

(continued)

Execution

1. *Start position.* Stand with the spine bent forward and the palms on the mat or as close to the mat as your flexibility allows, as shown. Walk the palms forward to Front Support as shown.

2. *Inhale.* Bend the elbows and lower the chest toward the mat. See the main muscle illustration.

3. *Exhale.* Straighten the elbows and raise the trunk to Front Support. Do two more push-ups (steps 2 and 3), and then walk the palms back as the hips flex to return to the start position. Repeat the entire sequence five times.

Targeted Muscles

Anterior spinal stabilizers: rectus abdominis, external oblique, internal oblique, transversus abdominis

Shoulder flexors: anterior deltoid, pectoralis major (clavicular), coracobrachialis, biceps brachii (long head)

Scapular abductors: serratus anterior, pectoralis minor

Elbow extensors: triceps brachii, anconeus

Accompanying Muscles

Spinal extensors and posterior spinal stabilizers: erector spinae

Hip extensors: gluteus maximus, hamstrings

Hip flexors: iliopsoas, rectus femoris

Knee extensors: quadriceps femoris

Shoulder extensors: latissimus dorsi, teres major, pectoralis major (sternal)

Technique Cues

- When walking out to Front Support in mid start position, swing one arm forward using the shoulder flexors, place it on the mat, and then shift the torso forward over the arm through use of the shoulder extensors. As the body weight shifts in front of this support hand, after the other arm swings forward, the shoulder flexors act to keep the chest lifted and the upper torso from lowering toward the mat.

- Keep the pelvis lifted to encourage use of the abdominals to prevent the lower back from arching, and use the hip flexors to prevent hip hyperextension due to gravity as the arms walk forward and the pelvis lowers.

- When you reach Front Support in the late start position, avoid the common error of leaving the buttocks lifted in the air. Use the hip extensors to bring the bottom of the pelvis down toward the mat as the abdominals lift (abdominal–hamstring force couple) so that the pelvis comes in line with the ankles and shoulders.

- As with Leg Pull Front (page 142), in Front Support focus on using the scapular abductors to keep the scapulae wide and the knee extensors to keep the knees straight to form a long line from the heels to the head.
- In step 2, keep the elbows close by the sides as eccentric contraction of the elbow extensors controls the bending of the elbows and eccentric contraction of the shoulder flexors controls the backward movement of the upper arms, resulting in the lowering of the chest toward the mat.
- In step 3, the elbow extensors straighten the elbows, and the shoulder flexors bring the upper arms forward to raise the chest back to Front Support.
- *Imagine.* Imagine that the legs, trunk, and head form a drawbridge that is lowered and raised with the arms, pivoting on the toes without altering the structural integrity of the strong bridge during steps 2 and 3.
- *Imagine.* When walking backward in step 3, think of lifting the pelvis up toward the ceiling like a drawbridge, keeping your abdominals scooped in throughout the movement. Then focus on using the hip extensors to pull down the sit bones to help bring the pelvis into place and stabilize it.

Exercise Notes

Push-Up shares some of the benefits of Leg Pull Front, including learning to maintain a neutral Front Support with skilled use of the abdominals and scapular abductors. However, Push-Up involves movement of the arms rather than the legs in Front Support. For many people, the weight of the body is sufficient to provide important strength benefits for the shoulder flexors and elbow extensors. The shoulder flexors are used to raise the arms to the front in everyday or sporting activities, while the elbow extensors are used in pushing and overhead lifting motions. Furthermore, the dynamic movement in and out of Front Support provides additional core challenges to achieve a coordinated transition from spinal flexion to extension and back to flexion. The initial position offers potential dynamic flexibility benefits for the hamstring muscles.

Modifications

If hamstring tightness prohibits placing the palms on the mat at the beginning of the exercise, bend the knees sufficiently to allow the body weight to be supported on the palms. As Front Support is approached, smoothly straighten the knees. Perform push-ups in this position before returning to the start position, again using bent knees when transitioning to standing.

If you are having difficulty achieving the desired positioning, just practice walking out to Front Support without adding the push-up and then back again.

SIDE EXERCISES FOR AN EFFECTIVE CORE

This chapter focuses on lateral flexion and rotation of the spine. Using lateral flexion and rotation is one way to place greater emphasis on the obliques versus the rectus abdominis. As described in chapter 2, the muscle fibers of the obliques are located more toward the sides of the trunk. These oblique muscles, particularly the internal oblique muscles, act with the transversus abdominis to protect the back and stabilize the core when the limbs move. Many athletic and recreational endeavors, such as swimming, kayaking, golf, throwing sports, and tennis, involve extensive use of the obliques. Improving your understanding, strength, and coordinated use of the obliques can enhance athletic performance and prevent back injuries. Therefore, include exercises from this chapter in every workout unless contraindicated for you.

The first three exercises require a sideways trunk position. This position changes the relationship of the trunk to the ground, so the lateral spinal flexors have to counter the effect of gravity. The obliques are key lateral spinal flexors. The quadratus lumborum and spinal extensors can also produce lateral flexion. Excessive contraction of the obliques combined with inadequate use of the spinal extensors will cause the trunk to round forward (spinal flexion) and flex laterally. Conversely, excessive contraction of the spinal extensors will cause the back to arch (spinal extension) and flex laterally. Therefore, finely coordinated contraction of the anterior and posterior muscles of the spine is required to achieve the desired position. This challenge is made more difficult by the fact that the spine is made up of many joints, with the lower back naturally curving opposite the upper back. Hence, side positions can be valuable practice for maintaining a neutral position of the pelvis and lower spine and learning the skill of bracing. Bracing can foster the transfer of core stabilization to many activities of daily living. Side Kick (page 150) and Side Kick Kneeling (page 152) use the lateral flexors as stabilizers while one leg swings. Side Bend (page 154) uses the lateral flexors as prime movers as the trunk is lowered and raised from a position of side support on one arm and the feet.

The remaining exercises use rotation. Spine Twist (page 158) and Saw (page 161) use the spinal rotators from a sitting position. Again, the obliques are emphasized, but coordinated use of the spinal extensors is essential to achieve the flat back position. Twist (page 164) adds rotation to Side Bend, a challenging combination of lateral flexion and rotation for those with adequate strength and skill. Corkscrew (page 168) and Hip Twist With Stretched Arms (page 171) emphasize rotation of the pelvis rather than rotation of the upper trunk. The pelvis is a vital link when transferring forces from and to the ground. Improving coordinated control of the pelvis is often neglected but highly needed. Note that these last two exercises are very advanced. Improper execution or a preexisting back condition could result in back injury. They should be attempted only after you have gained proficiency with related preparatory exercises to allow proper execution and only if your medical provider considers them appropriate for you.

Side Kick

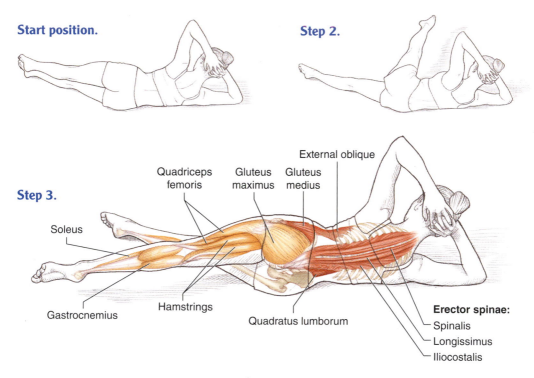

Start position.

Step 2.

Step 3.

External oblique

Quadriceps femoris

Gluteus maximus

Gluteus medius

Soleus

Gastrocnemius

Hamstrings

Quadratus lumborum

Erector spinae:
Spinalis
Longissimus
Iliocostalis

Execution

1. *Start position.* Lie on one side, with both legs slightly forward relative to the trunk and the feet gently pointed. Bend both elbows, interlace the fingers behind the head, and lift the head off the mat.

2. *Inhale.* Bring the top leg forward, slightly backward, and then, moving gently, forward just a little farther as shown.

3. *Exhale.* Bring the top leg backward, slightly forward, and then, moving gently, backward just a little farther. See the main muscle illustration. Repeat the sequence 10 times. Do the same on the opposite leg.

Targeted Muscles

Spinal lateral flexors and stabilizers: external oblique, internal oblique, quadratus lumborum, erector spinae (spinalis, longissimus, iliocostalis), semispinalis, deep posterior spinal group, rectus abdominis, transversus abdominis

Hip abductors: gluteus medius, gluteus minimus, tensor fasciae latae, sartorius

Accompanying Muscles

Hip flexors: iliopsoas, rectus femoris

Hip extensors: gluteus maximus, hamstrings

Knee extensors: quadriceps femoris

Ankle–foot plantar flexors: gastrocnemius, soleus

Technique Cues

- In the start position, use the spinal lateral flexors on the side closest to the mat to pull the pelvis up slightly toward the rib cage so the waist begins to lift off the mat. Attempt to maintain this distance between the pelvis and rib cage throughout the exercise.

- Use the hip abductors to keep the top leg parallel to the mat in steps 2 and 3; do not let it drop down. Use the hip flexors to bring the leg forward and the hip extensors to bring the leg back. Simultaneously the knee extensors keep the knee straight, and the ankle–foot plantar flexors point the foot.

- Emphasize using the spinal stabilizers to keep the body on its side and to limit the forward or backward rocking or rotating of the trunk, tilting of the pelvis, or arching of the back as the leg moves. In step 3, particularly focus on using adequate abdominal contraction and bringing the leg back only slightly to limit the amount of anterior pelvic tilt for safety and to maximize the dynamic stretch of the hip flexors.

- *Imagine.* Imagine the leg swinging forward freely at the hip joint, with a gentle recoil at the end of the range of movement before going farther in the same direction, and then swinging backward to repeat the same recoil action, with little movement of the trunk.

Exercise Notes

Side Kick is a valuable exercise for developing core stability. Lying on one side makes it difficult to maintain balance in a forward–backward direction because of the narrow base of support. The leg swing makes this balance challenge more difficult, making muscles on the sides, front, and back of the spine work in a coordinated manner to maintain equilibrium. If adequate stability of the spine and pelvis is maintained, Side Kick also offers dynamic flexibility benefits for the hamstrings and hip flexors. In this side-lying position, the hip abductors of the top leg have to work to prevent the leg from lowering because of gravity. Increased muscular endurance and tone in these muscles are desirable additional benefits.

Variations

Perform the exercise with the upper trunk lifted off the mat as you rest on the elbow as shown for greater challenge for the spinal lateral flexors, the scapular stabilizers, and balance. Flexing the foot (ankle–foot dorsiflexion) as the leg comes forward will emphasize the dynamic hamstring stretch. Reverse the breath pattern, with a percussive breath accompanying the double pulse in both directions.

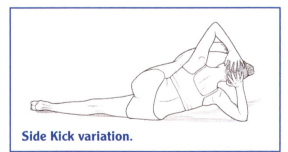

Side Kick variation.

Side Kick Kneeling

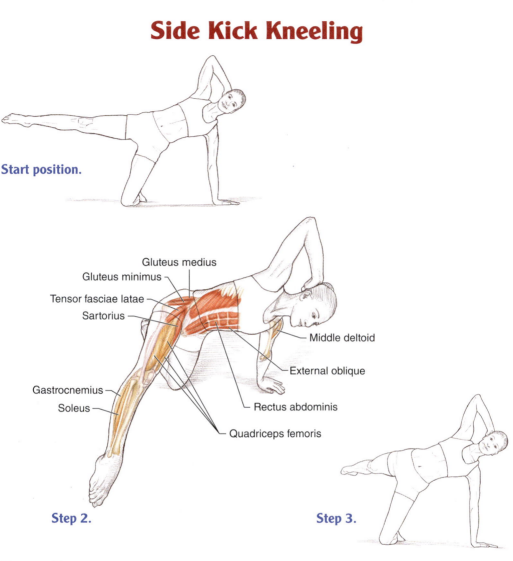

Start position.

Gluteus medius

Gluteus minimus

Tensor fasciae latae

Sartorius

Middle deltoid

External oblique

Gastrocnemius

Soleus

Rectus abdominis

Quadriceps femoris

Step 2.

Step 3.

Execution

1. *Start position.* Kneel and bend the trunk to the side. Place one palm on the mat, with the fingers pointing away from the knee. Place the other hand behind your head, with the elbow bent and pointing toward the ceiling. Lift the leg farthest from the support arm to about hip height.

2. *Inhale.* Bring the raised leg forward. See the main muscle illustration.

3. *Exhale.* Bring the raised leg backward as shown. Repeat the sequence five times. Do the same on the opposite leg.

Targeted Muscles

Spinal lateral flexors and stabilizers: external oblique, internal oblique, quadratus lumborum, erector spinae (spinalis, longissimus, iliocostalis), semispinalis, deep posterior spinal group, rectus abdominis, transversus abdominis

Hip abductors: gluteus medius, gluteus minimus, tensor fasciae latae, sartorius

Accompanying Muscles

Hip flexors: iliopsoas, rectus femoris

Hip extensors: gluteus maximus, hamstrings

Knee extensors: quadriceps femoris

Ankle–foot plantar flexors: gastrocnemius, soleus

Shoulder abductors: middle deltoid, supraspinatus

Scapular depressors: lower trapezius, serratus anterior (lower fibers)

Scapular abductors: serratus anterior

Elbow extensors: triceps brachii

Technique Cues

- Throughout the exercise, think of the body forming an arc from the head to the support knee. Press into the mat with the hand, and use the shoulder abductors to help lift the upper trunk, the spinal lateral flexors on the side of the body closest to the mat to lift the spine, and the hip abductors to lift the lower side of the pelvis, all to help form this arc.

- As you press into the mat, use the elbow extensors to keep the elbow straight while keeping the lower scapula down and reaching toward the mat with the use of the scapular depressors and abductors, particularly the serratus anterior.

- Maintain a long line of the raised leg as it swings, using the knee extensors to straighten the knee and the ankle–foot plantar flexors to point the foot.

- Focus on keeping the raised leg at the appropriate height by using the hip abductors while the hip flexors bring the leg forward and the hip extensors bring it slightly back.

- *Imagine.* Think of the body as an arched bridge, with the arm providing an upright support as the leg swings freely forward and backward without disrupting the strong bridge structure.

Exercise Notes

Side Kick Kneeling offers many of the same benefits as Side Kick (page 150), but it increases the stability challenge since you are supported by just one knee and one straight arm. It also increases the work of the spinal lateral flexors on the side closest to the mat, particularly the obliques, to maintain the side-arched position of the trunk. Last, it provides important practice for using the shoulder abductors and scapular stabilizers on the support arm, a skill that will be used in a much more difficult manner in the upcoming Side Bend (page 154) and Twist (page 164).

Variations

Perform the exercise with the support knee almost directly under the hip joint and the swinging leg held as high as possible to add greater challenge to the hip abductors. A double-leg pulse and the foot positioning and percussive breath pattern described in the Side Kick variations (page 151) can also be used.

Side Bend

Early start position.

Late start position.

Step 2.

Step 3.

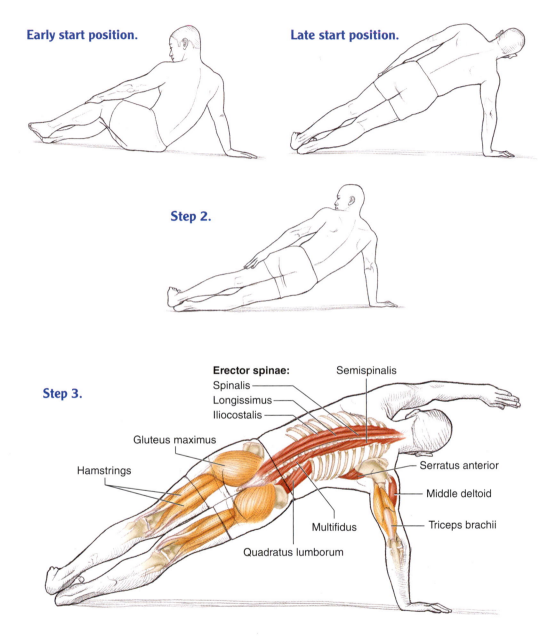

Erector spinae:
Spinalis
Longissimus
Iliocostalis

Semispinalis

Gluteus maximus

Hamstrings

Serratus anterior

Middle deltoid

Triceps brachii

Multifidus

Quadratus lumborum

Execution

1. *Start position.* Sit with the body rotated to the side, the weight supported by one arm, the lower side of the pelvis, and the lower foot. One palm is on the mat, with the fingers pointing away from the pelvis. The knees are bent, with the top hand resting on the side of the top knee as shown. From this position, lift the trunk up, straightening the knees and the upper arm while keeping the top arm close to the side of the body as shown.

2. *Inhale.* Turn the head toward the upper shoulder, and lower the lower part of the trunk until the lower calf comes in contact with the mat while the bottom arm remains straight as shown.

3. *Exhale.* Lift the trunk back up to the start position, and then bring the upper arm overhead, palm facing up and the head facing front. See the main muscle illustration. Repeat the sequence five times, and then bend the knees to lower to the early start position. Repeat the exercise on the opposite side.

Targeted Muscles

Spinal lateral flexors and stabilizers: external oblique, internal oblique, quadratus lumborum, erector spinae (spinalis, longissimus, iliocostalis), semispinalis, deep posterior spinal group (especially multifidus), rectus abdominis, transversus abdominis

Shoulder abductors: middle deltoid, supraspinatus, anterior deltoid, pectoralis major (clavicular)

Scapular depressors: lower trapezius, serratus anterior (lower fibers), pectoralis minor

Scapular abductors: serratus anterior, pectoralis minor

Accompanying Muscles

Hip extensors: gluteus maximus, hamstrings

Hip abductors: gluteus medius, gluteus minimus

Knee extensors: quadriceps femoris

Shoulder adductors: pectoralis major with latissimus dorsi

Elbow extensors: triceps brachii

Technique Cues

- In the last part of step 1 and in step 3, think of making an arc from the head to the support foot by pressing into the mat with the support hand and using the shoulder abductors to help lift the lower side of the upper trunk, the spinal lateral flexors to lift the lower side of the spine, and the hip abductors to lift the lower side of the pelvis.

(continued)

Side Bend   *(continued)*

- As you press into the mat, emphasize using the elbow extensors to keep the elbow straight while carefully avoiding elbow hyperextension. Simultaneously use the scapular depressors to keep the bottom of the scapula down and reach toward the mat with the scapular abductors, particularly the serratus anterior.

- In step 3, focus on arching the trunk and taking the top arm up and over the support arm, like water projecting out of a drinking fountain. To emphasize the lifted feeling, coordinate the peak of the arch of the upper torso with the peak of the arm movement overhead. The movement of the top arm is produced by concentric use of the shoulder abductors, followed by eccentric contraction of the shoulder adductors to control the lowering after the arm has passed vertical.

- In between steps 1 and 3, emphasize the lowering of the trunk in a smooth, controlled manner, using the same muscles described in the first cue, only now in an eccentric manner. Also, pay particular care to use the scapular depressors to prevent the support shoulder from rising toward the ear. Time the lowering of the top arm to return to the side of the body as the pelvis reaches its lowest point. Initially use the shoulder adductors and then the shoulder abductors eccentrically after the top arm passes vertical.

- *Imagine.* As the trunk rises and lowers, try to keep the body flat, as if moving between two parallel plates of glass. Use the knee extensors to keep the knees straight and the hip extensors to keep the hip joints extended, the thighs in line with the pelvis. The abdominals, spinal extensors, and other spinal stabilizers are used to maintain a flat back without the pelvis rotating or tilting either forward or backward.

Exercise Notes

Side Bend represents a very large jump in difficulty from Side Kick (page 150) and Side Kick Kneeling (page 152) in terms of lateral flexion, trunk stabilization, and shoulder use since just the feet and one arm support the body. This position makes this an excellent exercise for developing side trunk stability and muscular strength of the spinal lateral flexors. For many people, the biggest potential benefit is increased strength in the shoulder abductors and scapular stabilizers. In various phases of the exercise, gravity attempts to elevate or adduct the scapula. The scapular depressors, particularly the serratus anterior, must act to keep the scapula down and wide, abducted away from the spine, in its neutral position. If inadequate strength or coordination prevents you from doing this exercise with good form, you may experience shoulder discomfort or injury. Therefore, work in as small a range of motion as necessary to maintain good scapular mechanics, or modify the exercise.

Modification

Begin the exercise in the initial start position with only the bottom knee resting on the mat. Lift the trunk with the weight supported on one arm and the bottom knee rather than the feet.

Variations

Perform the exercise with the foot of the upper leg on the mat in front of the foot of the bottom leg as shown to provide a wider base of support and aid with balance. For an alternative breath pattern, lift on the inhale to the side plank position, with the top arm rising to shoulder height (T position). Exhale as you raise your pelvis and bring the arm overhead. Inhale to return to T position, and exhale to lower the pelvis until it is just above or slightly touches the mat.

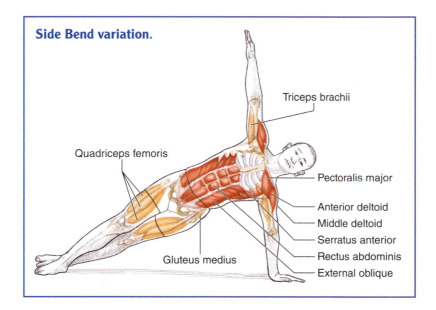

Side Bend variation.

Triceps brachii

Quadriceps femoris

Pectoralis major

Anterior deltoid

Middle deltoid

Serratus anterior

Gluteus medius

Rectus abdominis

External oblique

Spine Twist

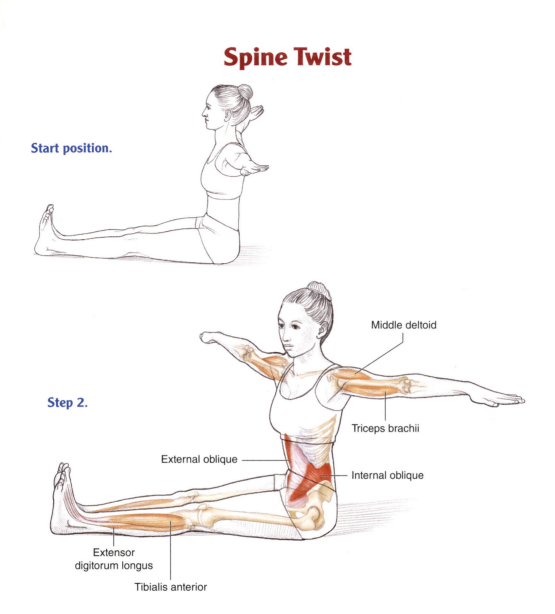

Start position.

Step 2.

Middle deltoid

Triceps brachii

External oblique

Internal oblique

Extensor
digitorum longus

Tibialis anterior

Execution

1. *Start position.* Sit with the legs together and outstretched to the front, feet flexed (ankle–foot dorsiflexion). The arms are straight and out to the sides, reaching slightly back, at shoulder height with the palms facing down.

2. *Exhale.* Rotate the upper trunk to one side and then slightly farther in that same direction. See the main muscle illustration.

3. *Inhale.* Rotate the upper trunk back to center (start position).

4. *Exhale.* Rotate the upper trunk to the opposite side and then slightly farther in that same direction.

5. *Inhale.* Rotate the trunk back to center (start position). Repeat the sequence 5 times on each side, 10 times in total.

Targeted Muscles

Spinal rotators: external oblique, internal oblique, erector spinae (longissimus, iliocostalis), semispinalis, deep posterior spinal group (especially multifidus)

Accompanying Muscles

Anterior spinal stabilizer: transversus abdominis

Ankle–foot dorsiflexors: tibialis anterior, extensor digitorum longus

Shoulder abductors: middle deltoid, supraspinatus

Elbow extensors: triceps brachii

Scapular adductors: trapezius, rhomboids

Technique Cues

- In the start position, focus on pulling the abdominal wall in and up as you think of lifting up from the base of the lower back to maintain a vertical position of the spine throughout the exercise.
- Emphasize rotating above the pelvis so that the pelvis remains stationary and facing forward as the spinal rotators twist the spine from the lower back to the base of the head.
- Reach the arms to the sides, with the shoulder abductors keeping the arms at shoulder height while the elbow extensors straighten the elbows and help create the desired long line. Simultaneously pull your shoulder blades together very slightly with the scapular adductors. Maintain this position of the arms relative to the upper trunk as you rotate.
- *Imagine.* Imagine the spine spiraling up as it twists so that it feels as if your head is getting closer to the ceiling as you rotate.

Exercise Notes

Spine Twist shares some of the same benefits as Spine Twist Supine (page 62). However, the vertical position of the spine in Spine Twist provides additional value because you are in a similar position to one used in many everyday activities and athletic activities, such as golf and tennis. Also, keeping the body upright against gravity challenges the trunk musculature in a slightly different way. Learning to use the powerhouse rather than the shoulders for rotation is key to this exercise and fundamental for creating optimal athletic performance and preventing common injuries to the back.

(continued)

Spine Twist   *(continued)*

Sitting trunk rotation. When you rotate to the right while in a sitting position, the left external and right internal obliques generally act as the prime movers. However, if they acted alone, they also would make the torso bend forward since they are spinal flexors as well as rotators. Appropriate activation of the spinal extensors is necessary to keep the spine vertical. As shown in the illustration, these extensors, particularly the right longissimus, right iliocostalis, left semispinalis, and left multifidus, also assist with right rotation of the trunk. Appropriate cocontraction of these and other muscles allows the spine to rotate without bending forward or arching backward.

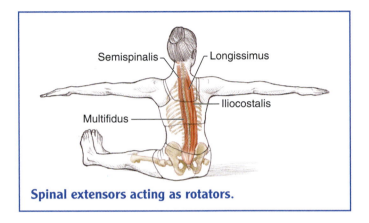

Spinal extensors acting as rotators.

Variations

This exercise can also be performed with the arms directly out to the sides, the scapulae in a neutral position, and the shoulders externally rotated with the palms facing up. In addition, a percussive breath can accompany the double pulse in each direction.

Saw

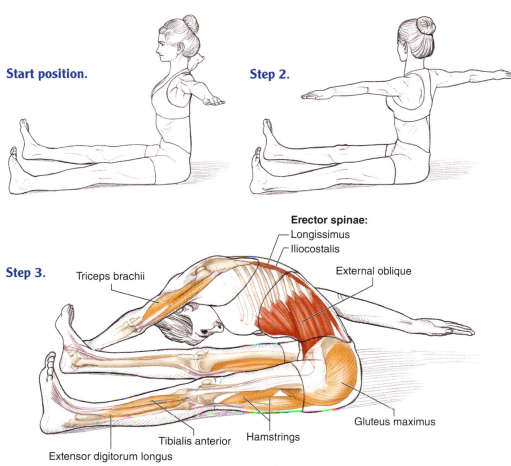

Start position.

Step 2.

Step 3.

Erector spinae:
Longissimus
Iliocostalis

External oblique

Triceps brachii

Gluteus maximus

Hamstrings

Tibialis anterior

Extensor digitorum longus

Execution

1. *Start position.* Sit with the trunk upright, legs slightly wider than shoulder-width apart, knees straight, and feet flexed (ankle–foot dorsiflexion). Hold the arms out to the sides at shoulder height, reaching slightly back, with elbows straight and palms facing down.

2. *Inhale.* Rotate the upper trunk to one side as shown, and then bring the head and upper spine forward and downward so that the hand reaches to the outside of the opposite foot, if your current flexibility allows, while the back arm internally rotates and reaches back and slightly upward.

3. *Exhale.* Very gently reach the arm slightly farther forward with three consecutive sawlike motions. See the main muscle illustration. Bring the trunk up to vertical, and then rotate back to the start position.

4. *Inhale.* Rotate the upper trunk to the opposite side, and repeat the rest of step 2 on this new side.

5. *Exhale.* Perform step 3 on this new side. Repeat the sequence 5 times on each side, 10 times in total.

(continued)

161

Saw *(continued)*

Targeted Muscles

Spinal rotators: external oblique, internal oblique, erector spinae (longissimus, iliocostalis), semispinalis, deep posterior spinal group

Spinal extensors: erector spinae (spinalis, longissimus, iliocostalis), semispinalis, deep posterior spinal group

Accompanying Muscles

Anterior spinal stabilizer: transversus abdominis

Hip extensors: gluteus maximus, hamstrings

Ankle–foot dorsiflexors: tibialis anterior, extensor digitorum longus

Shoulder abductors: middle deltoid, supraspinatus

Shoulder flexors: anterior deltoid, pectoralis major (clavicular)

Shoulder extensors: latissimus dorsi, teres major

Elbow extensors: triceps brachii

Scapular adductors: trapezius, rhomboids

Technique Cues

- In step 1 and the first part of step 2 and step 4, apply the technique cues described for Spine Twist (page 158), particularly focusing on the coordinated contraction of the abdominals and spinal extensors to rotate the upper trunk while it remains vertical.

- In the late part of step 2 and step 4, smoothly roll the spine down, controlling it by an eccentric contraction of the spinal extensors. The pelvis remains facing forward, with both sit bones firmly in contact with the mat.

- As the hand reaches forward in step 3 and step 5, think of gently lengthening the spine slightly farther with each sawlike motion. Avoid using large bounces, which could be injurious to the spine. Simultaneously, gently draw in the abdominal wall to avoid an anterior tilt of the pelvis.

- Focus on reaching the arms in opposite directions in steps 2 through 5, particularly as the front arm moves forward and the shoulder flexors become key in preventing it from lowering toward the mat and as the back arm internally rotates, reaching and lifting to the back with the use of the shoulder extensors.

- During the roll-up in step 3 and step 5, continue to use the abdominals to pull in the abdominal wall. Simultaneously use the spinal extensors to return the spine to vertical by stacking one vertebra at a time on the sacrum, from the lumbar spine upward.

- When rotating the upper trunk back to center at the end of steps 3 and 5, focus on reaching the head up toward the ceiling to encourage slight cocontraction of the spinal extensors while the obliques primarily affect the rotation.

- Simultaneously return the arms to their start position. Think of reaching the arms out to the sides, with the little fingers pressing slightly back to encourage activation of the scapular adductors as the shoulder abductors work to keep the arms at shoulder height and the elbow extensors work to keep the elbows straight.

- *Imagine.* During the rotation of the trunk, imagine the upper spine is like a screwdriver, maintaining a vertical position as it twists to tighten or loosen a screw on the top of a table. The legs and pelvis act like the table, staying stationary as only the screw and screwdriver move.

Exercise Notes

As with Spine Twist (page 158), Saw is beneficial for learning to rotate the trunk by using the core muscles while maintaining a vertical position. However, in Saw, the trunk also moves off vertical, which offers valuable practice for applying spinal articulation in a rotated position when the spine rolls down and then back up. Furthermore, the position with the spine flexed forward provides a dynamic stretch for the lower back and hamstrings from an off-center position.

Variation

Change the start position so the arms are directly out to the sides, the scapulae in neutral position, and the shoulders externally rotated so that the palms are forward. To deemphasize primarily flexing the upper back and place greater emphasis on stretching the hamstrings, hold the thoracic spine in extension while placing greater emphasis on flexing at the hip

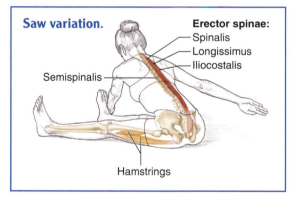

Saw variation.

Semispinalis

Erector spinae:
Spinalis
Longissimus
Iliocostalis

Hamstrings

joint, with the sit bones reaching back as the spine reaches forward as shown. In this variation, thoracic and hip extension, not a gradual articulation of the spine, are emphasized on the return to vertical (step 3 and step 5).

Twist

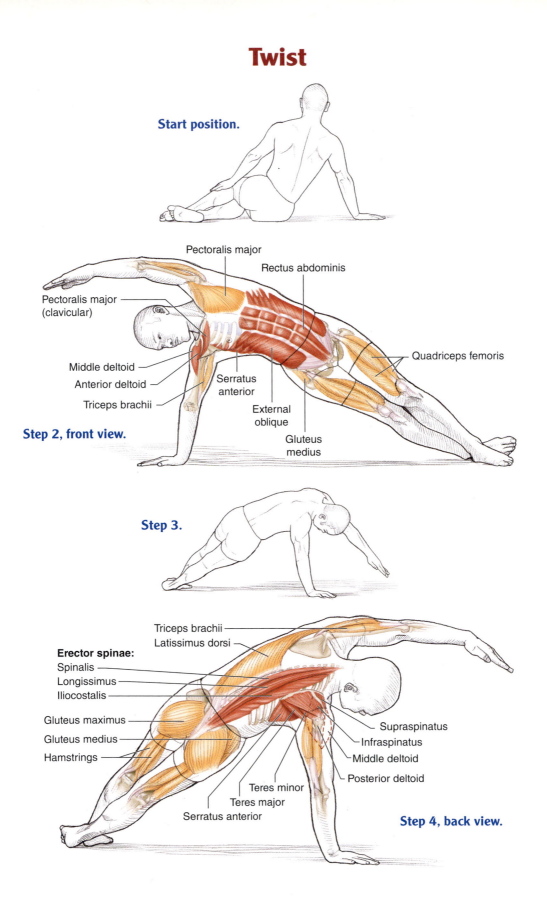

Start position.

Pectoralis major

Rectus abdominis

Pectoralis major
(clavicular)

Middle deltoid

Anterior deltoid

Triceps brachii

Serratus
anterior

External
oblique

Gluteus
medius

Quadriceps femoris

Step 2, front view.

Step 3.

Triceps brachii

Latissimus dorsi

Erector spinae:

Spinalis

Longissimus

Iliocostalis

Gluteus maximus

Gluteus medius

Hamstrings

Supraspinatus

Infraspinatus

Middle deltoid

Posterior deltoid

Teres minor

Teres major

Serratus anterior

Step 4, back view.

Execution

1. *Start position.* Sit with the body rotated to the side. Support your weight on one arm (palm on the mat with the fingers pointing away from the pelvis), the lower side of the pelvis, and the feet (foot of the top leg in front of the other foot). Knees are bent, with the top hand resting on the side of the top knee.

2. *Inhale.* Lift the trunk toward the ceiling as the legs straighten and the top arm rises overhead as shown. See the front view of the muscle illustration. The head can face forward or slightly down.

3. *Exhale.* Rotate the upper trunk toward the mat as shown.

4. *Inhale.* Rotate back to the position of step 2, as shown in the back view of the muscle illustration.

5. *Exhale.* Bend the knees and lower the trunk and top arm toward the start position, stopping with the pelvis just above the mat, if good form can be maintained. If necessary, lower to the point at which the mat provides a brief moment of support. Repeat the sequence five times. Do the same on the opposite side.

Targeted Muscles

Spinal lateral flexors and rotators: external oblique, internal oblique, quadratus lumborum, erector spinae (spinalis, longissimus, iliocostalis), semispinalis, deep posterior spinal group, rectus abdominis, iliopsoas

Shoulder abductors: middle deltoid, supraspinatus, anterior deltoid, pectoralis major (clavicular)

Shoulder horizontal abductors: infraspinatus, teres minor, posterior deltoid, middle deltoid, teres major, latissimus dorsi

Scapular depressors: lower trapezius, serratus anterior (lower fibers), pectoralis minor

Scapular abductors: serratus anterior, pectoralis minor

Accompanying Muscles

Anterior spinal stabilizer: transversus abdominis

Hip extensors: gluteus maximus, hamstrings

Hip abductors: gluteus medius, gluteus minimus

Knee extensors: quadriceps femoris

Knee flexors: hamstrings

Shoulder adductors: pectoralis major with latissimus dorsi

Elbow extensors: triceps brachii

(continued)

Twist *(continued)*

Technique Cues

- See the technique cues for Side Bend (page 154) for a more detailed description of the muscles working in step 2.

- In step 2, press the support arm into the mat and use the shoulder abductors, spinal lateral flexors, and hip abductors to lift the lower side of the body and create an arc from the head to the feet. The hip extensors and knee extensors straighten the legs and bring them in line with the pelvis.

- As the pelvis is lifting, smoothly raise the top arm overhead, initially using the shoulder abductors to lift the arm. After the arm passes vertical, eccentrically use the shoulder adductors to prevent gravity from lowering the arm too far. Use the scapular abductors of the bottom arm to keep the scapula in its desired wide position and to counter the tendency of gravity to bring the scapula toward the spine.

- In step 3, use the spinal rotators to bring the upper trunk to face down toward the mat. Use the obliques to maximize the rotation as the erector spinae work eccentrically to control the rotary effects of gravity. In this rotated end position, the shoulder flexors and horizontal abductors hold the free arm up, preventing it from falling toward the mat or across the body.

- In step 4, use the erector spinae to rotate the trunk in the opposite direction, while the abdominals assist with the rotation and keep the lower back from arching.

- In step 5, eccentrically use the shoulder abductors, spinal lateral flexors, and hip abductors of the lower side of the body to control the body as it lowers toward the mat. The knee flexors slowly bend the knees. At this point, the scapular depressors of the support arm prevent undesired lifting of the scapulae, while the shoulder adductors begin and the shoulder abductors continue eccentrically to control the lowering of the top arm.

- Throughout the exercise, provide controlled support with the bottom arm. The elbow extensors keep the elbow straight. Various shoulder and scapular muscles come into play as the trunk changes its relationship to the support arm and gravity, with the shoulder horizontal abductors playing a particularly key role eccentrically in step 3 and concentrically in step 4.

- *Imagine.* Visualize a dolphin breaching the water, arcing and then spiraling as it reenters the water. Then reverse this visualization as if playing a film backward.

Exercise Notes

Think of Twist as adding rotation to the challenges of Side Bend (page 154). Twist should not be performed until proficiency with Side Bend has been achieved. Although Twist is not shown in *Return to Life Through Contrology*, it is commonly performed in a variety of ways by different schools of Pilates training. The version described here reflects a clear direct progression from Side Bend. Twist is a very challenging exercise that recruits a large number of muscles in different phases of the movement. Two key potential benefits it offers relate to rotational core stability, as well as strength and complex coordination of vital muscles of the shoulder complex. In Twist, one shoulder not only supports a great deal of the body weight but also moves through a large range of motion while bearing this weight. Therefore, excellent mechanics of the shoulder are required when performing Twist to reap the potential benefits and prevent potentially serious injury.

Variations

Twist can also be performed by bringing the top arm to the T position, aligned with the shoulders in steps 2 and 4, rather than overhead. As the top arm reaches under the body, lift the hips high to maximize spinal rotation and create a pyramid shape, with the legs straight and the thoracic spine extended as much as hamstring flexibility allows. An even more challenging variation is to keep the knees straight throughout, including during the lifting and lowering phases (steps 2 and 5).

Corkscrew (Corkscrew Advanced)

Start position.

Step 2.

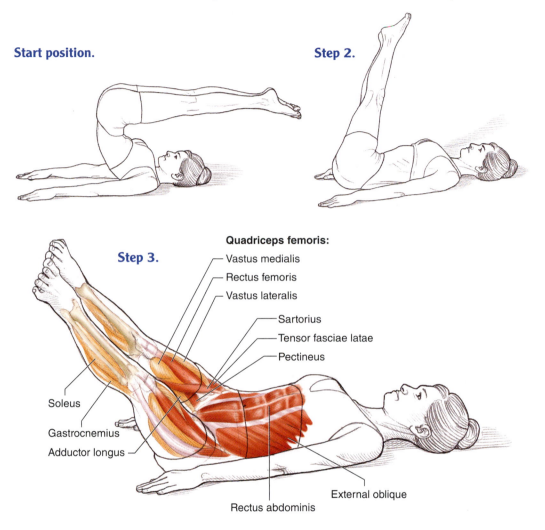

Step 3.

Quadriceps femoris:

Vastus medialis

Rectus femoris

Vastus lateralis

Sartorius

Tensor fasciae latae

Pectineus

Soleus

Gastrocnemius

Adductor longus

External oblique

Rectus abdominis

Execution

1. *Start position.* Perform Rollover With Legs Spread (page 112) to get into position with the legs overhead and approximately parallel to the mat.

2. *Exhale.* Twist the lower trunk so that one side of the body comes closer to the mat. Both legs shift to that side as the trunk and legs begin to lower as shown.

3. *Inhale.* Circle the legs down on that side, across center, up on the opposite side as shown in the main muscle illustration, and then overhead to the center start position.

4. *Exhale.* Shift the lower trunk and both legs to the side opposite that used in step 2.

5. *Inhale.* Circle the legs down that side, through the center, and up the other side, returning overhead to the center start position. Repeat the sequence three times on each side, six times in total, alternating sides with each exhale.

Targeted Muscles

Spinal flexors and anterior rotators: rectus abdominis, external oblique, internal oblique

Hip flexors: iliopsoas, rectus femoris, sartorius, tensor fasciae latae, pectineus

Accompanying Muscles

Anterior spinal stabilizer: transversus abdominis

Spinal extensors and posterior rotators: erector spinae

Hip extensors: gluteus maximus, hamstrings

Hip adductors: adductor longus, adductor brevis, adductor magnus, gracilis

Knee extensors: quadriceps femoris

Ankle–foot plantar flexors: gastrocnemius, soleus

Shoulder extensors: latissimus dorsi, teres major, posterior deltoid

Technique Cues

- Apply the technique cues described for Rollover With Legs Spread (page 112), including using the abdominals to posteriorly tilt the pelvis and sequentially flex the spine as you roll up and over in step 1.

- As the lower trunk rotates in steps 2 through 5, allow the legs to shift with the pelvis so that the legs maintain their same relationship to the midline of the front of the pelvis.

- In steps 3 and 5, the hip extensors start the movement as the legs circle down, but in the lower arc of the circle, the hip flexors work eccentrically to control the legs as they lower and then concentrically to help begin the up circle to the other side. Take particular care to make the circles small enough, and use adequate abdominal contraction to prevent the lower back from arching or the pelvis from anteriorly tilting.

- As the legs circle, think of pressing down into the mat with the arms at the appropriate time so the shoulder extensors can help raise the lower torso or keep both shoulders in full contact with the mat. The spinal rotation occurs below the armpits, with complex use of the spinal rotators, particularly the abdominals, concentrically working to produce rotation of the spine and pelvis and then eccentrically working to control the rotation in different phases of the movement.

- Throughout the exercise, think of gently squeezing the inner thighs together to activate the hip adductors while the knee extensors keep the legs straight and the ankle–foot plantar flexors point the feet to create a long, arrowlike leg line. As the legs circle to the sides, the hip adductors of the bottom leg help keep the legs lifted to the desired height.

- *Imagine.* Imagine drawing a circle with your feet, using a very strong core to help the legs maintain their appropriate relationship to the moving pelvis.

(continued)

Corkscrew (Corkscrew Advanced)   *(continued)*

Exercise Notes

Corkscrew incorporates the challenges of spinal articulation and core stability of Rollover With Legs Spread (page 112), but it markedly increases the difficulty since you must circle the legs to the sides rather than just move them up and down to the front. Bringing the legs and pelvis to one side tends to cause the whole trunk to move to that side. But complex rotational stabilization keeps the shoulders and upper back in full contact with the mat as the lower trunk rotates without the lower back excessively arching or the ribs jutting forward. In addition to developing stabilization skills, the overhead position of Corkscrew can provide dynamic flexibility benefits for the hamstrings and lower back.

Although Corkscrew offers many potential benefits, the combination of rotation and flexion or extension of the spine puts the body in a very vulnerable position. In addition, this exercise requires weighted flexion of the upper back and neck, previously seen in Rollover With Legs Spread. Perform this exercise only if it is appropriate for you and after you have achieved proficiency with Spine Twist Supine (page 62) and Rollover With Legs Spread.

Modifications

Begin and end each circle with the legs at 90 degrees (vertical) and the back of the pelvis flat on the mat rather than with the legs overhead and the pelvis off the mat. Bend the knees slightly if the hamstrings are tight or to make stabilization easier. When stabilization improves, progress to the overhead position if it is appropriate for you.

After progressing to the overhead position, if the hamstrings or lower back are tight, bend the knees slightly or allow the feet to be as far from the mat as necessary to facilitate supporting the body weight primarily on the upper back and shoulders, not the neck.

Variation

This exercise can also be done with an inhale for the initial part of the circle (upper section) and an exhale for the remainder of the circle (lower section) to encourage activation of the deep abdominal muscles to help keep the lower back pressed against the mat and prevent the common error of allowing the back to arch as the legs move down and away from the center. The illustrations show inadequate and adequate abdominal stabilization.

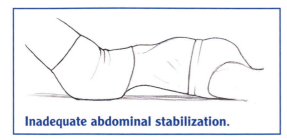

Inadequate abdominal stabilization.

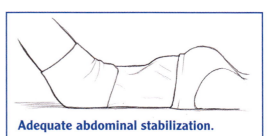

Adequate abdominal stabilization.

Hip Twist With Stretched Arms
(Hip Circles Prep)

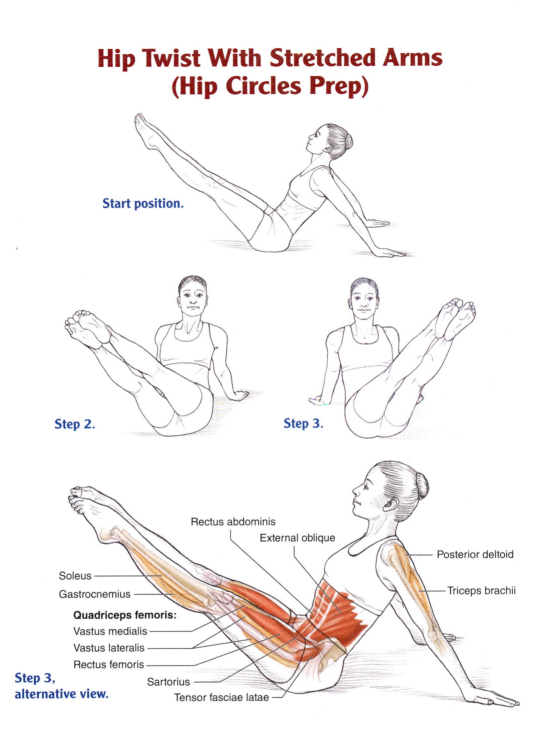

Start position.

Step 2.

Step 3.

Rectus abdominis

External oblique

Posterior deltoid

Soleus

Gastrocnemius

Quadriceps femoris:

Vastus medialis

Vastus lateralis

Rectus femoris

Sartorius

Tensor fasciae latae

Triceps brachii

Step 3,
alternative view.

Execution

1. *Start position.* Start rocked back on the sit bones to balance, with the arms behind the trunk and the palms of the hands flat on the mat, fingers pointing back. Hold the legs in a V position.

2. *Exhale.* Rotate the pelvis, shifting both legs to one side of the body as shown, down on that side, and across center.

(continued)

3. *Inhale.* Continue the circle, bringing the legs up the opposite side as shown, rotating the pelvis to that side (see the main muscle illustration), and then bringing the legs and pelvis back to the center start position.

4. *Exhale.* Rotate the pelvis and bring both legs to the side of the body opposite that in step 2, down on that side, and across center.

5. *Inhale.* Continue the circle, bringing the legs up the side opposite that of step 3, rotating the pelvis to that side and then bringing the legs and pelvis back to the center start position. Repeat the sequence three times on each side, six times in total, alternating sides with each exhale.

Targeted Muscles

Spinal flexors and anterior rotators: rectus abdominis, external oblique, internal oblique

Hip flexors: iliopsoas, rectus femoris, sartorius, tensor fasciae latae, pectineus

Accompanying Muscles

Anterior spinal stabilizer: transversus abdominis

Spinal extensors and posterior rotators: erector spinae

Hip adductors: adductor longus, adductor brevis, adductor magnus, gracilis

Knee extensors: quadriceps femoris

Ankle–foot plantar flexors: gastrocnemius, soleus

Shoulder extensors: latissimus dorsi, teres major, posterior deltoid

Scapular depressors: lower trapezius, serratus anterior (lower fibers)

Elbow extensors: triceps brachii

Technique Cues

• In the start position, allow the pelvis to posteriorly tilt, but use the shoulder extensors and upper spinal extensors to lift the upper back. Use the scapular depressors to pull the scapulae down slightly to limit the natural elevation of the scapulae that accompanies the end range of shoulder extension.

• Use the spinal flexors and anterior rotators to twist the lower trunk while the shoulders remain directly forward. The feet maintain their alignment with the midline of the pelvis throughout the circling in steps 2 through 5.

• Take extra care to use adequate abdominal stabilization, and keep the circles small enough so your lower back does not arch and your pelvis does not tilt anteriorly.

- Throughout the exercise, think of gently pulling the inner thighs together to activate the hip adductors. The knee extensors keep the legs straight, and the ankle–foot plantar flexors point the feet so a long, arrowlike leg line is maintained.
- *Imagine.* Imagine that your feet are holding a laser beam that must keep its light shining on the midline of the pelvis, extending up from the pubic symphysis. Although the legs move up or down relative to the pelvis as they circle, the pelvis and legs always face the same direction as the pelvis shifts from side to side.

Exercise Notes

Hip Twist With Stretched Arms provides similar potential benefits to those offered by Corkscrew (page 168), especially in terms of complex rotational stabilization. However, the challenge increases since the more upright position requires greater balance and puts the hip flexors in a shortened position, so greater strength is required to support the legs. Although potentially offering valuable benefits in terms of hip flexor strength, as well as dynamic hamstring and shoulder flexor flexibility, this is a very advanced exercise that requires excellent form to reduce risk to the lower back. Perform it only if not contraindicated for your back, and initially use the modifications, if needed.

Modifications

If your hamstrings are tight or you have difficulty keeping the pelvis and lower back stable, perform the movement with the knees slightly bent or while leaning farther back, supported on the forearms.

Variation

The breathing pattern can be reversed; inhale as the pelvis rotates and the legs are taken to one side, and then exhale as the legs circle down and around to promote core stability.

EXTENSIONS FOR A STRONG BACK

This chapter focuses on improving the strength, muscular endurance, and skilled activation of the spinal extensors. Prior chapters emphasized use of the abdominals primarily to produce spinal flexion or use of the abdominals with assistance from the spinal extensors to produce lateral flexion or rotation. This chapter emphasizes use of the spinal extensors to produce or maintain spinal hyperextension, while the abdominals function as stabilizers to reduce the potentially injurious forces borne by the lower back. This use of spinal extension is vital for maintaining muscle balance because so many Pilates exercises emphasize spinal flexion. In addition, adequate strength and endurance of the spinal extensors may reduce the risk of osteoporosis and lower back injury. However, spinal hyperextension is also a common mechanism for producing injury to the lower back. Optimal technique and careful progression from less demanding to more demanding exercises are essential to enhance potential benefits and reduce the risks of these exercises.

The first exercise will help you work on technique. Cat Stretch (page 176) is a relatively simple and well-supported way to practice using the spinal extensors to create hyperextension with greater emphasis on the upper back, while the abdominals cocontract to limit excessive hyperextension in the lower back. One-Leg Kick (page 178) uses this cocontraction to keep the upper trunk totally still in hyperextension while one leg moves at a time. The challenge is to maintain core stability with the spine in hyperextension. Double Kick (page 181) uses this skilled abdominal cocontraction while the spinal extensors act as prime movers, producing substantial movement of the spine instead of primarily acting to stabilize the spine. Swimming (page 184) requires that the spine be maintained in slight hyperextension while the opposite arm and leg repetitively lift and lower. This represents a novel exercise for maintaining stability in that the limbs are moving in opposition.

The last two exercises require maintenance of the spine and hips in hyperextension while the trunk rocks forward and backward in space. In the first of these exercises, Rocking (page 187), the hands hold the feet, which is helpful for maintaining the almost fixed arch of the spine as the body moves. In contrast, in Swan Dive (page 190) the arms and legs are free, and the spinal extensors are even more critical in maintaining the desired arch of the back. Both exercises are very advanced. If you improperly execute the exercises or have a preexisting back condition, it could result in injury to your back. These exercises should be attempted only after you have achieved proficiency with related preparatory exercises, if you experience no back discomfort, and if they are not contraindicated for your back.

Cat Stretch

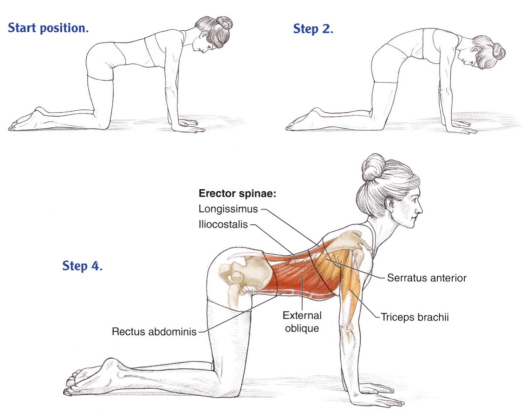

Start position.

Step 2.

Step 4.

Erector spinae:
Longissimus
Iliocostalis

Serratus anterior

Triceps brachii

External
oblique

Rectus abdominis

Execution

1. *Start position.* Start on the hands and knees, with the arms directly under the shoulders and the knees directly under the hip joints. The pelvis and spine are in a neutral position.
2. *Exhale.* Posteriorly tilt the pelvis and round the spine as shown.
3. *Inhale.* Return to the start position.
4. *Exhale.* Extend the upper spine. See the main muscle illustration.
5. *Inhale.* Return to the start position. Repeat the entire sequence five times.

Targeted Muscles

Spinal extensors: erector spinae (spinalis, longissimus, iliocostalis), semispinalis, deep posterior spinal group

Spinal flexors: rectus abdominis, external oblique, internal oblique

Accompanying Muscles

Anterior spinal stabilizer: transversus abdominis

Hip extensors: gluteus maximus, hamstrings

Shoulder flexors: anterior deltoid, pectoralis major (clavicular)

Shoulder extensors: latissimus dorsi, teres major, pectoralis major (sternal)

Scapular abductors: serratus anterior

Elbow extensors: triceps brachii

Technique Cues

- In the start position, pull up the lower attachment of the abdominals onto the pelvis while drawing the abdominal wall slightly toward the spine, just enough to create a neutral position of the pelvis and spine.
- In step 2, draw in the abdominals farther as they are used to flex the spine. At the same time, gently pull the tailbone (coccyx) under as you use the hip extensors and abdominals to posteriorly tilt the pelvis.
- Press your hands into the mat, using the shoulder flexors to lift the upper trunk slightly toward the ceiling as the scapular abductors allow the scapulae to separate.
- In step 3, smoothly return to the start position, emphasizing eccentric use of the abdominal muscles.
- In step 4, use the spinal extensors as you reach the head and upper back out and up toward the ceiling. The abdominals simultaneously limit anterior tilting of the pelvis and excessive arching in the lumbar region of the spine. Press your hands into the mat, using the scapular abductors to keep the scapulae wide and the shoulder extensors to help raise the upper trunk into the arched position.
- *Imagine.* Imagine a hand placed on your lower back. Focus on rounding the lower spine to press into the hand to emphasize flexing the lumbar spine in step 2, and then focus on reaching the upper spine away from the hand in step 4.

Exercise Notes

Although Cat Stretch is not included in *Return to Life Through Contrology,* it is an excellent exercise for practicing the skills needed for the more demanding exercises that follow. The benefit of this exercise is not so much strengthening of the spinal extensors but detailed activation of the spinal extensors with appropriate cocontraction of the abdominals. The trunk has four-point support. From this position, the spinal extensors are activated in step 4 to arch the back, emphasizing extension of the thoracic spine, while cocontraction of the abdominals limits the magnitude of anteriorly tilting the pelvis. This use of the abdominals is essential for protecting the lower back in exercises that are more complex and involve greater forces. Moving the spine in the opposite direction in step 2 is an opportunity to further practice activating the abdominals to emphasize rounding the lower back (flexion). This position provides a dynamic stretch for the spinal extensors and offers a valuable interlude between exercises that focus on using the back extensors.

One-Leg Kick (Single-Leg Kick)

Start position.

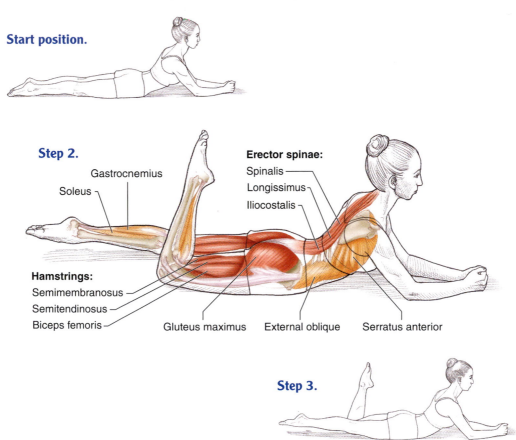

Step 2.

Gastrocnemius

Soleus

Erector spinae:
Spinalis
Longissimus
Iliocostalis

Hamstrings:
Semimembranosus
Semitendinosus
Biceps femoris

Gluteus maximus   External oblique   Serratus anterior

Step 3.

Execution

1. *Start position.* Lie prone, resting on the forearms with the upper trunk lifted off the mat. Position the forearms so the upper arms form an approximately 90-degree angle with the trunk. Hands are on the mat next to each other, fists clenched. Legs rest on the mat straight to the back and together, feet gently pointed.

2. *Inhale.* Lift both legs about 2 inches (5 cm) off the mat. Bend one knee so that the heel comes toward the buttocks with a brisk dynamic. See the main muscle illustration.

3. *Exhale.* With the same brisk dynamic, straighten the bent knee as you bend the opposite knee so that the opposite heel comes toward the buttocks as shown. Repeat the sequence 10 times on each leg, 20 times in total.

Targeted Muscles

Spinal extensors: erector spinae (spinalis, longissimus, iliocostalis), semispinalis, deep posterior spinal group

Hip extensors: gluteus maximus, hamstrings (semimembranosus, semitendinosus, biceps femoris)

Accompanying Muscles

Anterior spinal stabilizers: transversus abdominis, internal oblique, external oblique, rectus abdominis

Knee flexors: hamstrings

Knee extensors: quadriceps femoris

Ankle–foot plantar flexors: gastrocnemius, soleus

Shoulder extensors: latissimus dorsi, teres major, pectoralis major (sternal)

Scapular depressors: lower trapezius, serratus anterior (lower fibers)

Scapular abductors: serratus anterior

Technique Cues

- Throughout the exercise, firmly contract the abdominals. Focus on pulling the lower abdominals up to limit the anterior tilt of the pelvis. (This is described more fully in Back Extension Prone, page 66.)
- Press the forearms into the mat as you lift your upper back toward the ceiling to encourage use of the shoulder extensors and upper spinal extensors. Use the scapular depressors to pull the scapulae down slightly while using the scapular abductors to keep them wide.
- In step 2, use the hip extensors to lift the legs only to a height at which an anterior tilt of the pelvis can be avoided. Throughout the exercise, maintain this height while keeping the legs close together. Use the ankle–foot plantar flexors to keep the feet pointed.
- In the later part of step 2, use the knee flexors to bend one knee briskly, but keep the force and range of motion small enough to avoid any knee discomfort.
- In step 3, the knee extensors are used briefly to begin straightening the bent knee, followed by an eccentric contraction of the knee flexors to control the straightening of the knee produced primarily by gravity. The knee flexors of the opposite knee bend that knee.
- *Imagine.* Isolate the movement of the lower legs to the knee joints. The rest of the body remains stable, with the trunk held in a smooth arc like that of a sea lion pressing up from its flippers.

(continued)

One-Leg Kick (Single-Leg Kick)   *(continued)*

Exercise Notes

One-Leg Kick is a valuable core stability exercise that emphasizes the spinal extensors keeping the spine off the mat with additional support provided by the arms. The leg movements challenge this stability. The action of the legs also potentially provides hip extensor muscle tone and endurance benefits, particularly for the hamstring muscles that keep the legs lifted off the mat and bend the knees. Full flexion of the knee can provide a dynamic stretch for the quadriceps femoris muscle group, which is often tight. The abdominal muscles play a vital stabilizing role by limiting the anterior tilt of the pelvis and preventing excessive hyperextension in the lowest portion of the back, a stabilizing skill used with increasingly demanding exercises in this chapter.

Modification

If you experience back discomfort, limit the amount of spinal extension by putting the elbows farther forward or resting the forehead on the hands.

Variation

Perform the exercise with the elbows directly under the shoulders to increase spinal extension and further challenge the spinal extensors and abdominal stabilizers.

Double Kick (Double-Leg Kick)

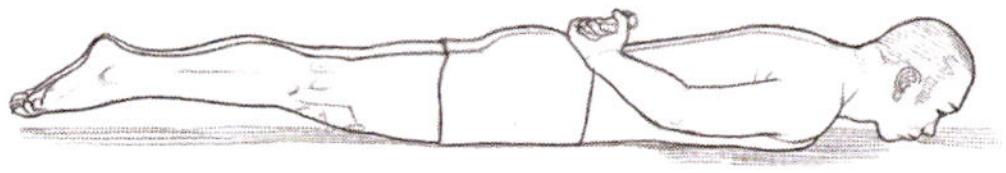

Start position.

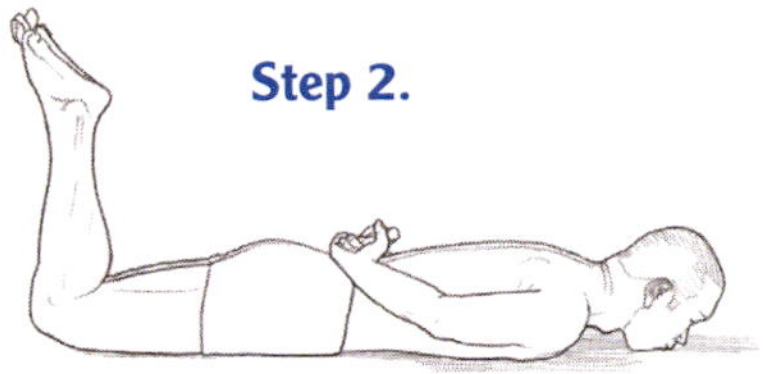

Step 2.

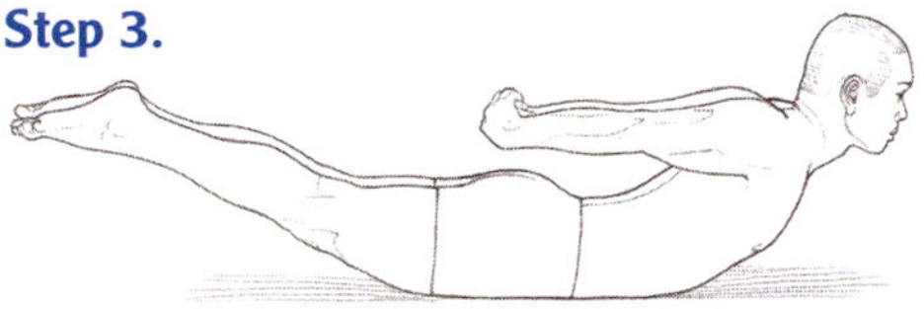

Step 3.

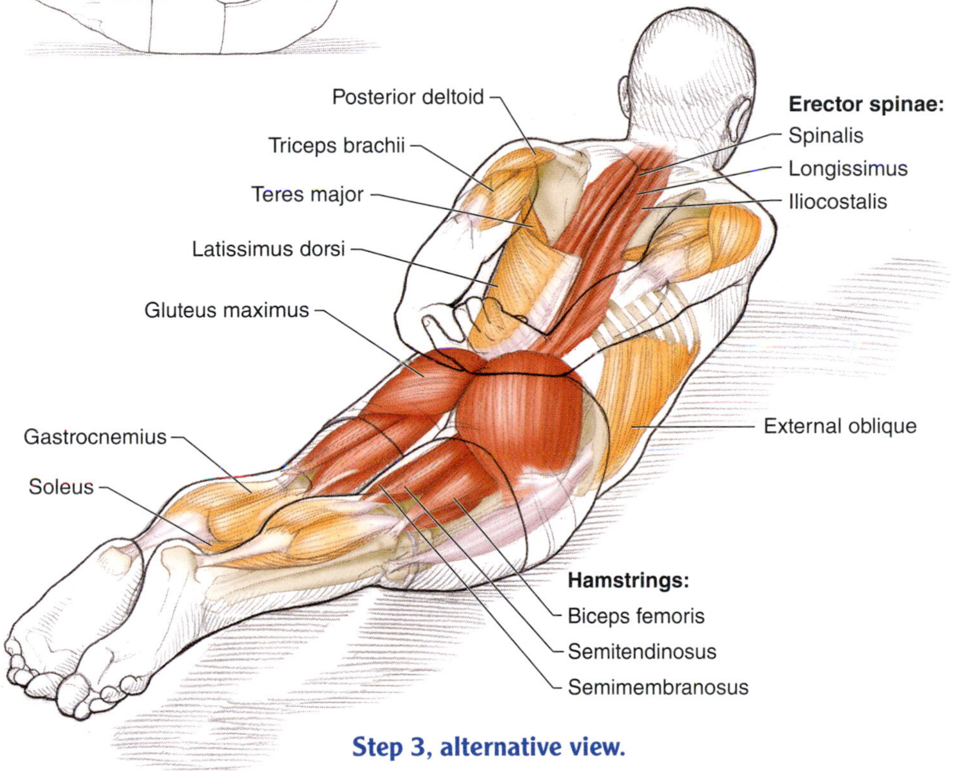

Posterior deltoid

Triceps brachii

Teres major

Latissimus dorsi

Gluteus maximus

Gastrocnemius

Soleus

Erector spinae:
Spinalis
Longissimus
Iliocostalis

External oblique

Hamstrings:
Biceps femoris
Semitendinosus
Semimembranosus

Step 3, alternative view.

Execution

1. *Start position.* Lie prone, chin resting on the mat. Bend the elbows, with the fingers of one hand grasping the opposite hand and the backs of the hands resting on the sacrum. Lift both legs about 1 inch (2 cm) off the mat, knees remaining straight and feet gently pointed.

2. *Exhale.* Gently bend both knees, bringing the heels toward the buttocks as shown with a brisk dynamic.

3. *Inhale.* Raise the chest off the mat, straighten the elbows, and reach the hands back toward the feet as you straighten the knees and reach the heels back and up toward the ceiling as shown. See the main muscle illustration. Return to the start position. Repeat the sequence six times.

(continued)

Targeted Muscles

Spinal extensors: erector spinae (spinalis, longissimus, iliocostalis), semispinalis, deep posterior spinal group

Hip extensors: gluteus maximus, hamstrings (semimembranosus, semitendinosus, biceps femoris)

Accompanying Muscles

Anterior spinal stabilizers: transversus abdominis, internal oblique, external oblique, rectus abdominis

Hip adductors: adductor longus, adductor brevis, adductor magnus, gracilis

Knee flexors: hamstrings

Knee extensors: quadriceps femoris

Ankle–foot plantar flexors: gastrocnemius, soleus

Shoulder extensors: latissimus dorsi, teres major, posterior deltoid

Scapular depressors: lower trapezius, serratus anterior (lower fibers)

Elbow flexors: biceps brachii, brachialis

Elbow extensors: triceps brachii

Technique Cues

- Throughout the exercise, focus on pulling the lower abdominals up and in to limit the anterior tilt of the pelvis.
- In the start position, use the hip extensors to lift the legs slightly off the mat and the ankle–foot plantar flexors to point the feet.
- In step 2, keep the knees off the mat as the knee flexors gently bend the knees. Keep the ankles together and feet pointed, but allow the knees to separate slightly if needed. This will allow the natural inward motion of the lower leg that accompanies knee flexion to occur without producing undue stress on the knees.
- After the knee extensors begin to straighten the legs in step 3, focus on using the hip adductors to pull the legs slightly together, and emphasize pointing the feet as the legs reach out in space to create a long line.
- As the legs straighten in step 3, smoothly raise the chest off the mat, using the spinal extensors to arch the spine sequentially from top to bottom. Simultaneously use the scapular depressors to pull the scapulae down slightly as the shoulder extensors raise the arms back and the elbow extensors straighten the elbows.

- As you return to the start position, use an eccentric contraction of the spinal extensors to smoothly control the upper trunk as it lowers, and bend the elbows with the elbow flexors.
- *Imagine.* Imagine the trunk and legs are a bow, with the arms acting like the bowstring. Pulling the string (arms) back results in a greater arc of the bow without disrupting its integrity.

Exercise Notes

Double Kick is closely related to One-Leg Kick (page 178). However, because the arms are not used for support and the back and legs are raised repetitively, Double Kick provides a more effective stimulus for improving strength and endurance of the spinal extensors. Lifting both legs also increases the difficulty for the abdominal muscles to maintain trunk stability. This exercise offers a dynamic stretch for the knee extensors for some people and shoulder flexors for many people. Shoulder flexor tightness is common and can contribute to the postural problem of rolled shoulders.

Variation

Start the exercise with one side of your face resting on the mat to avoid the neck hyperextension that comes from having the chin on the mat. As the spine arches, rotate the head to center, keeping the head in line with the arc of the trunk. As the chest lowers, bring the other side of the face to rest on the mat.

Swimming

Start position.

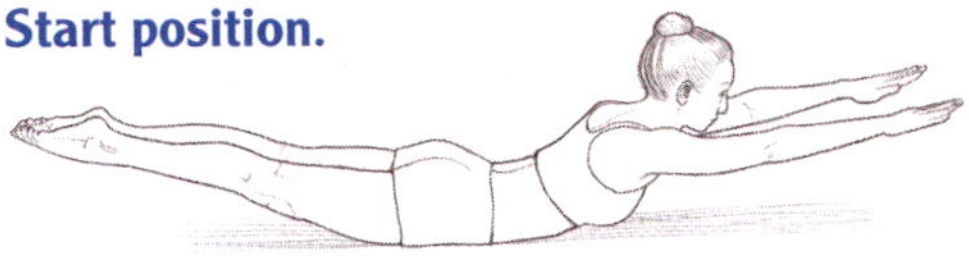

Step 2.

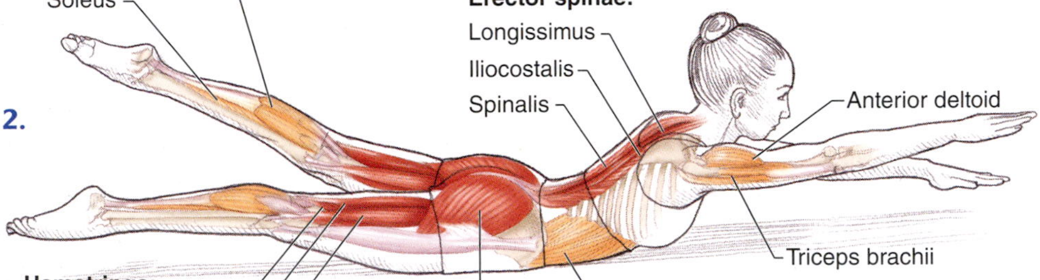

Gastrocnemius
Soleus

Erector spinae:
Longissimus
Iliocostalis
Spinalis

Anterior deltoid

Triceps brachii

Hamstrings:
Semimembranosus
Semitendinosus
Biceps femoris

External oblique

Gluteus maximus

Execution

1. *Start position.* Lie prone with the arms straight overhead and the palms facing down. Raise the chest, both arms, and both legs slightly off the mat. Knees are straight, feet gently pointed.

2. Raise the right arm and left leg as shown in the main muscle illustration.

3. Raise the left arm and right leg as the opposite limbs return to their start position. Continue for 10 breath cycles, alternating sides in a brisk but smooth manner. This exercise is presented in *Return to Life Through Contrology* without a set breath pattern and with instructions to breathe naturally.

Targeted Muscles

Spinal extensors and rotators: erector spinae (spinalis, longissimus, iliocostalis), semispinalis, deep posterior spinal group

Hip extensors: gluteus maximus, hamstrings (semimembranosus, semitendinosus, biceps femoris)

Accompanying Muscles

Anterior spinal stabilizers: transversus abdominis, internal oblique, external oblique, rectus abdominis

Hip flexors: iliopsoas, rectus femoris

Knee extensors: quadriceps femoris

Ankle–foot plantar flexors: gastrocnemius, soleus

Shoulder flexors: anterior deltoid, pectoralis major (clavicular)

Shoulder extensors: latissimus dorsi, teres major, pectoralis major (sternal)

Scapular depressors: lower trapezius, serratus anterior (lower fibers)

Elbow extensors: triceps brachii

Technique Cues

- Throughout the entire exercise, pull the lower abdominals up and in to limit the anterior tilt of the pelvis.

- In step 1, use the spinal extensors to lift the upper back as you raise the chest off the mat and the hip extensors to raise the legs. Simultaneously, use the scapular depressors to pull the scapulae down slightly to avoid excessive elevation while the shoulder flexors keep the arms off the mat.

- In steps 2 and 3, think of reaching the limbs out long and in opposite directions. The elbow extensors keep the elbow straight, while the knee extensors keep the knee straight, and the ankle–foot plantar flexors keep the foot pointed. While maintaining this reach, carefully coordinated actions between the shoulder flexors and shoulder extensors and the hip extensors and hip flexors produce the small but quick up and down movements of opposite limbs.

- *Imagine.* As the name of the exercise suggests, the action of the limbs can be likened to the flutter kick used when swimming. Imagine that your pelvis and lower back are supported by a kickboard, remaining lifted and stable as both the legs and arms perform a movement similar to the flutter kick.

Exercise Notes

Swimming is a valuable stability exercise that emphasizes the spinal extensors but with a different approach. While the spinal extensors actively contract to hold the spine off the mat, movement of one leg and one arm on opposite sides of the body occurs in the same direction. This type of limb movement is an important aspect of motor development and is used in many essential movements, such as walking and running.

Spinal rotation with opposite limb movement. As the left leg lifts higher, it will tend to make the lower trunk rotate to the left; when the right arm lifts higher, it will tend to make the upper trunk rotate to the right. To keep the trunk in the desired stationary position, you must call into play the rotational actions of the spinal

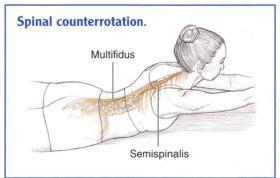

Spinal counterrotation.

Multifidus

Semispinalis

(continued)

Swimming   *(continued)*

extensors such as the left lumbar multifidus, with its action of right lumbar rotation, and the right semispinalis, with its action of left thoracic rotation. (See the illustration.) Both counter the spinal rotation that tends to accompany the movements of the limbs. Since the erector spinae produces rotation to the same side, opposite the direction of rotation produced by the multifidus and semispinalis, components of the erector spinae also work on the opposite side. Therefore, Swimming can develop trunk rotational stability. For some people, the action of the legs also provides potential benefits in terms of hip extensor muscle tone and endurance.

Variation

This exercise can also be performed using an inhale for five changes and an exhale for the next five changes. This is reminiscent of the breath pattern used in Hundred (page 78).

Rocking

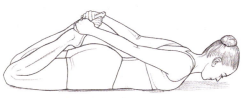

Early start position.

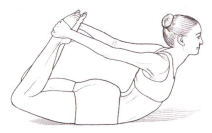

Late start position.

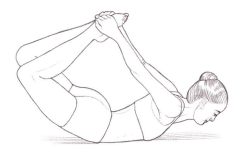

Step 2.

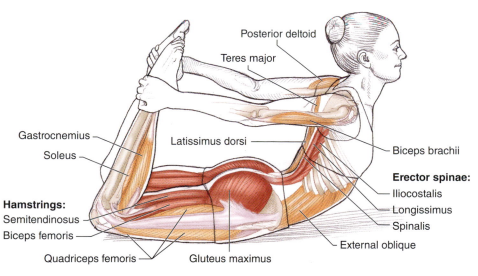

Posterior deltoid

Teres major

Gastrocnemius

Soleus

Latissimus dorsi

Biceps brachii

Erector spinae:
Iliocostalis
Longissimus
Spinalis

Hamstrings:
Semitendinosus
Biceps femoris

Quadriceps femoris

Gluteus maximus

External oblique

Step 3.

(continued)

Execution

1. *Start position.* Lie prone with the knees bent and close together, each hand grasping the foot on the same side of the body as shown. Raise the head, chest, and knees off the mat as shown.

2. *Inhale.* Rock the body forward as shown.

3. *Exhale.* Rock the body back as shown in the main muscle illustration. Repeat the sequence 10 times.

Targeted Muscles

Spinal extensors: erector spinae (spinalis, longissimus, iliocostalis), semispinalis, deep posterior spinal group

Hip extensors: gluteus maximus, hamstrings (semimembranosus, semitendinosus, biceps femoris)

Accompanying Muscles

Anterior spinal stabilizers: transversus abdominis, internal oblique, external oblique, rectus abdominis

Knee extensors: quadriceps femoris

Shoulder extensors: latissimus dorsi, teres major, posterior deltoid

Scapular depressors: lower trapezius, serratus anterior (lower fibers)

Elbow flexors: biceps brachii, brachialis

Technique Cues

- Throughout the exercise, maintain abdominal support, and limit the anterior tilt of the pelvis to a pain-free range.

- In the late start position, use the spinal extensors to arch the back as you lift the chest off the mat and the hip extensors raise the knees off the mat. Use the knee extensors to press the feet away from the buttocks and into the hands so the arms act to raise the upper trunk slightly higher off the mat.

- To begin forward rocking in step 2, use the hip extensors to lift the knees a little higher off the mat and the shoulder extensors to pull the feet up and forward. The elbow flexors assist with this pulling motion, but ideally the knee extensors prevent visible bending of the elbows.

- In step 3, think of the opposite motion. The feet go down and back as the spinal extensors work with greater intensity to lift the upper trunk against gravity.

- *Imagine.* Imagine that the head, trunk, and thighs form an arc, like the base of a rocking chair. As the chair rocks forward, the weight transfers onto the front of the arc (represented by the upper chest) while the back of the arc (represented by the thighs) rises farther off the mat. Conversely, when the chair rocks back, the weight shifts onto the back of the arc (thighs) while the front of the arc (upper chest) lifts higher off the ground.

Exercise Notes

Rocking shares the goal of exercises such as Rolling Back (page 100)—maintain the trunk in the same shape while it rolls through space. However, unlike Rolling Back, in Rocking the spine is maintained in a position of extension rather than flexion. Maintaining an arched position of the trunk requires highly skilled use of many muscles, including the spinal extensors and hip extensors. It also requires skilled use of the abdominals to reduce stress on the lower back. This exercise should be done only after proficiency has been gained in the exercises described earlier in this chapter. Even if proper technique is used, because of the high level of spinal hyperextension inherent in this exercise, it is not appropriate for many people. Although it provides strong benefits for back extensor endurance and core stability for appropriate people, it should not be performed if you experience back discomfort or if this degree of extension is contraindicated for your back. The extreme position used in this exercise also provides dynamic flexibility benefits for the shoulder flexors, hip flexors, and spinal flexors.

Swan Dive

Start position.

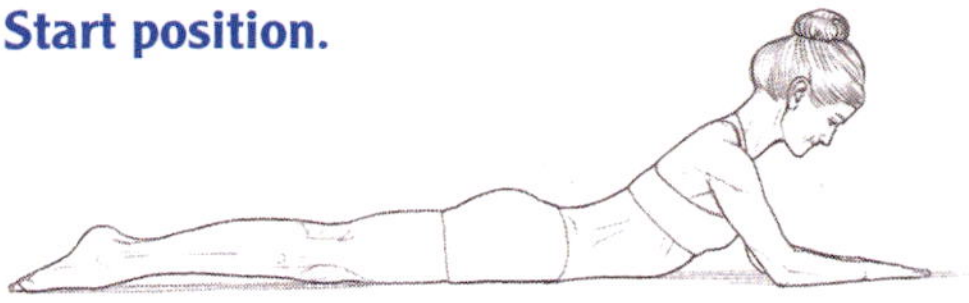

Step 2.

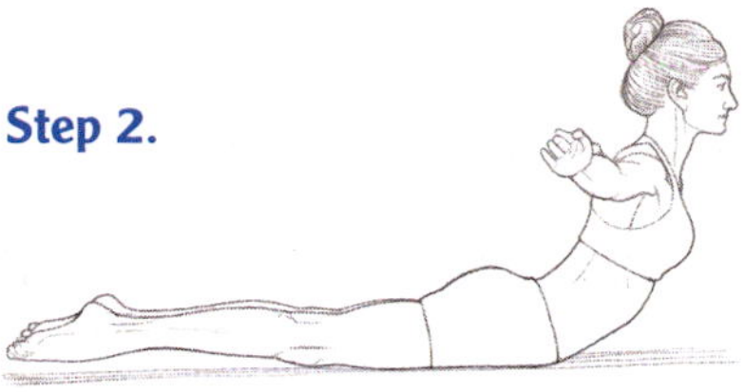

Step 2, alternative view.

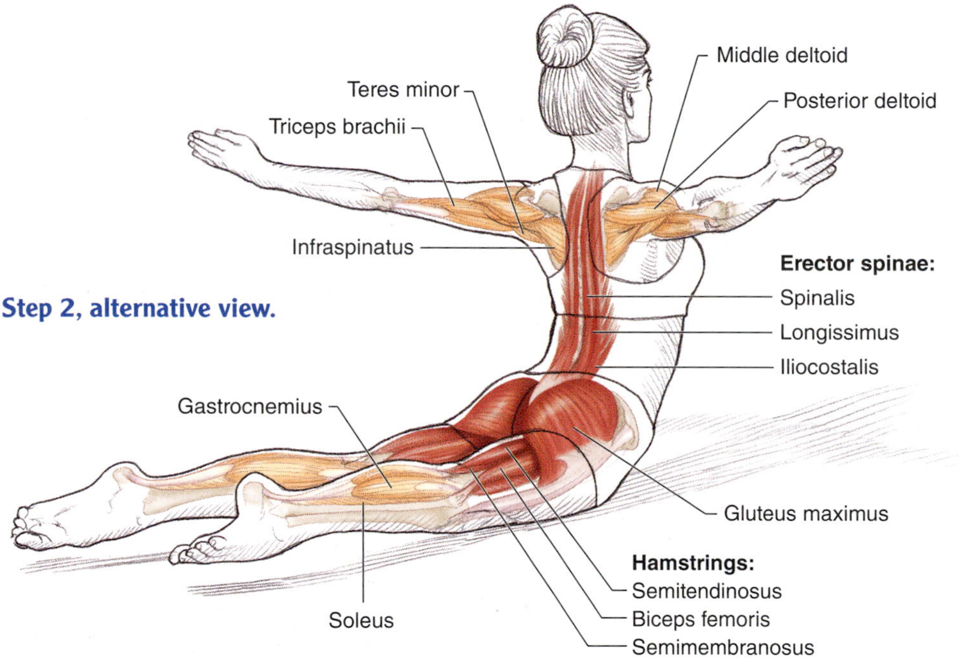

Teres minor
Triceps brachii
Infraspinatus

Middle deltoid
Posterior deltoid

Erector spinae:
Spinalis
Longissimus
Iliocostalis

Gastrocnemius

Gluteus maximus

Hamstrings:
Semitendinosus
Biceps femoris
Semimembranosus

Soleus

Step 3.

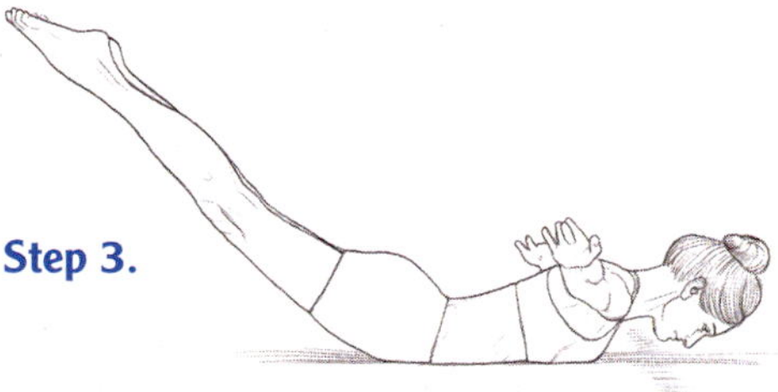

Execution

1. *Start position.* Lie prone, resting on the forearms with the upper trunk lifted off the mat. Place the elbows wider than and in front of the shoulders. Hands are next to each other. Legs rest on the mat straight to the back and close together, feet gently pointed.

2. *Inhale.* Lift the chest higher off the mat as you straighten the elbows and raise the arms out to the sides at shoulder height. At the same time, raise both legs off the mat. See the main muscle illustration.

3. *Exhale.* Rock the body forward as shown.

4. *Inhale.* Rock the body back to the lifted position of step 2. Repeat the sequence five times, rocking forward on the exhale and back on the inhale.

Targeted Muscles

Spinal extensors: erector spinae (spinalis, longissimus, iliocostalis), semispinalis, deep posterior spinal group

Hip extensors: gluteus maximus, hamstrings (semimembranosus, semitendinosus, biceps femoris)

Accompanying Muscles

Anterior spinal stabilizers: transversus abdominis, internal oblique, external oblique, rectus abdominis

Knee flexors: hamstrings

Ankle–foot plantar flexors: gastrocnemius, soleus

Shoulder horizontal abductors: infraspinatus, teres minor, posterior deltoid, middle deltoid

Scapular adductors: trapezius, rhomboids

Elbow extensors: triceps brachii

Technique Cues

- Throughout the exercise, maintain abdominal support, and limit the degree of the anterior tilt of the pelvis to a pain-free range.
- In step 2, use the spinal extensors to lift the upper back as you raise the chest off the mat and the hip extensors raise the legs.
- Use the shoulder horizontal abductors to lift the upper arms toward the ceiling and then back while the scapular adductors pull the scapulae together slightly as the elbow extensors straighten the elbows in step 2.
- In step 3, use the hip extensors to lift the legs higher off the mat, shifting the body weight farther forward so that the chest lowers closer to the mat.
- In step 4, think of the opposite motion—lifting the back higher off the mat with the back extensors as the legs lower closer to the mat but do not touch the mat.
- *Imagine.* As in Rocking (page 187), imagine that the head, trunk, and thighs form an arc like the base of a rocking chair, which rocks forward and back without flattening out. In Swan Dive, also imagine that your feet are being pulled toward the ceiling with a strong pulley in step 3 and that you are about to dive backward as the back comes up in step 4.

(continued)

Swan Dive   *(continued)*

Exercise Notes

Swan Dive increases muscle tone and endurance in the spinal extensors and, secondarily, in the hip extensors. Swan Dive shares with Rocking (page 187) the goal of maintaining the trunk in a position of extension as the body rocks forward and backward in space, but it offers a greater challenge because the arms do not help maintain this desired shape. Maintaining an arched position of the trunk requires highly skilled use of many core muscles, including appropriate activation of the spinal extensors in conjunction with the abdominals to reduce stress on the lower back while allowing hyperextension to occur. This exercise should be done only after proficiency has been gained in easier exercises. Even if proper technique is used, because of the high level of spinal hyperextension inherent in this exercise, it is not appropriate for many people. This exercise should not be done if contraindicated for your back. Even if it is deemed appropriate for your back, start with the modification, or use a small range of motion to reduce the risk of injury. The extreme position used in this exercise can also provide dynamic flexibility benefits for the hip flexors and spinal flexors.

Modification

To modify this exercise, keep the hands on the mat, extend the elbows partway or fully in step 2 to help lift the chest off the mat, and then bend the elbows in step 3 to help lower the chest.

Variation

This exercise can also be performed with the arms reaching overhead in step 2 instead of to the side and then remaining overhead as the body rocks, as shown in the illustrations. Maintaining this overhead position increases the challenge to the back extensors and may help you maintain a long arch as the body rocks forward and back.

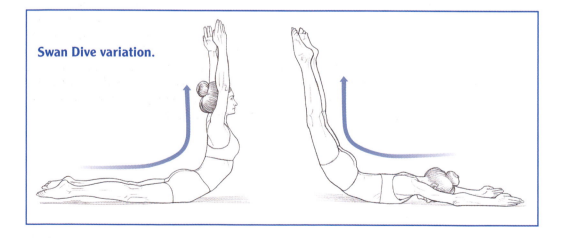

Swan Dive variation.

CUSTOMIZING YOUR PILATES PROGRAM

It is time to practice! Consistent practice is essential to reap the rewards of Pilates, and a well-structured program is key to maximizing gains from each session. You must consider many factors when customizing a program to your needs. Certain factors may change daily, while others remain consistent. Factors to be aware of are body type, past injuries, medical restrictions, age, gender, fitness level, and movement skills. Choose exercises wisely to maximize benefits and minimize the risk of injury.

There are different approaches to structuring a Pilates program. Joseph Pilates had a very specific sequence of the exercises he devised, a sequence still used by some people today. Other approaches have only a remote resemblance to Joseph Pilates' classic sequencing. It is particularly challenging to apply standard scientific principles of program design to a full-body Pilates mat program because so many of the exercises center on the *powerhouse,* the core of Pilates. However, structure is important to promote muscle balance, logical progression, and flow and continuity; in addition, structure offers an environment for creativity.

An important issue to consider is whether the program has a bias toward muscular strength or endurance. A program with an endurance bias will entail relatively high repetitions with lower resistance. (In mat work, resistance is provided by body weight and gravity only, unless small apparatus such as circles and bands are introduced.) In contrast, a strength-based program will use fewer repetitions of a particular exercise, but the load on the muscle will be greater, and the muscle that is worked to the point of fatigue must be allowed to recover for 2 or 3 minutes before being worked again.

The frequency and duration of a session are influenced by many factors, including your current fitness level, skill level, health, and schedule. When starting, it is generally recommended that you do 2 or 3 workouts of 20 to 60 minutes each per week. As you become more proficient, you can perform longer workouts, up to 90 minutes, more frequently. Remember, it is preferable to do a short session than no session at all. If you have limited time, are working hard, or are traveling, don't forgo your routine, just shorten it.

The sample programs shown in tables 10.1 (page 194), 10.2 (page 195), and 10.3 (page 196) use a sequencing that will encourage the development of muscular strength for some exercises and muscular endurance for others. Realize that certain Pilates exercises are designed primarily to develop important coordination skills, such as spinal articulation and core stability. The overload to the muscles in these exercises is simply insufficient to offer much potential strength benefit, and so these exercises can be readily interspersed between exercises that have more of a strength bias to offer active recovery time.

Table 10.1   Fundamental Pilates Program

Exercise	Page number	Level	Repetitions	Comments
Pelvic Curl	52	Fundamental	5	
Chest Lift	54	Fundamental	10	
Leg Lift Supine	56	Fundamental	5 each leg	Consecutive
Spine Twist Supine	62	Fundamental	5 each side	Alternating
Leg Lift Side	58	Fundamental	10 each side	Consecutive
Back Extension Prone	66	Fundamental	5	
One-Leg Circle	70	Fundamental	5 each leg	Alternating
Hundred	78	Intermediate	10 breath cycles	Use modification
Rolling Back	100	Fundamental	10	
Spine Stretch	98	Fundamental	5	
Shoulder Bridge	128	Intermediate	5 each leg	Use modification Consecutive
One-Leg Stretch	82	Fundamental	5 each leg	Alternating
Saw	161	Intermediate	5 each side	Alternating
Spine Twist	158	Intermediate	5 each side	Alternating
Side Kick	150	Fundamental	10 each leg	Consecutive
One-Leg Kick	178	Intermediate	10 each leg	Alternating
Cat Stretch	176	Fundamental	5	
Leg Pull Front	142	Intermediate	5 each leg	Use modification Alternating
Swimming	184	Intermediate	10 breath cycles	
Seal	102	Intermediate	5	Use modification

The programs in tables 10.1, 10.2, and 10.3 incorporate elements from each chapter: foundation, abdominal work, spinal articulation, bridging, sides of the body, and back extension. It is good to begin an exercise session with a general warm-up that includes movements to increase the internal body temperature and moderately elevate the heart rate, such as brisk walking or calisthenics. Follow the general warm-up with a specific warm-up of foundation movements described in chapter 4. Think of the specific warm-up as a series of movements that prepare you for the specific movement demands of the workout that follows. The warm-up prepares not only the body but also the mind. It offers an opportunity to transfer the focus from outside to inside, to bring awareness to the work and set the tone for the session.

Abdominal work is an important part of the program and a key element for a strong and well-functioning powerhouse. Abdominal work is complemented by spinal articulation. In *Return to Life Through Contrology,* Joseph Pilates wrote, "If your spine is inflexible at 30, you are old; if it is completely flexible at 60, you are young" (page 27). Bridging exercises,

Table 10.2 Intermediate Pilates Program

Exercise	Page number	Level	Repetitions	Comments
Pelvic Curl	52	Fundamental	5	
Chest Lift	54	Fundamental	10	
Leg Lift Supine	56	Fundamental	5 each leg	Consecutive
Spine Twist Supine	62	Fundamental	5 each side	Alternating
Leg Lift Side	58	Fundamental	10	Both exercises on same side; switch sides and repeat
Leg Pull Side	60	Fundamental	10	
Chest Lift With Rotation	64	Fundamental	5 each side	Alternating
Back Extension Prone	66	Fundamental	5	
One-Leg Circle	70	Fundamental	5 each leg	Alternating
Hundred	78	Intermediate	10 breath cycles	Use modification
Roll-Up	73	Intermediate	5	
Spine Stretch	98	Fundamental	5	
Rolling Back	100	Fundamental	10	
Shoulder Bridge	128	Intermediate	5 each leg	Consecutive
One-Leg Stretch	82	Fundamental	5 each leg	Alternating
Double-Leg Stretch	87	Intermediate	10	
Rocker With Open Legs	108	Intermediate	5	
Saw	161	Intermediate	5 each side	Alternating
Spine Twist	158	Intermediate	5 each side	Alternating
Rollover With Legs Spread	112	Advanced	6	Use modification
One-Leg Kick	178	Intermediate	10 each leg	Alternating
Side Kick	150	Fundamental	10 each leg	Consecutive
Double Kick	181	Intermediate	10	
Cat Stretch	176	Fundamental	5	
Leg Pull Front	142	Intermediate	5 each leg	Alternating
Swimming	184	Intermediate	10 breath cycles	
Side Kick Kneeling	152	Intermediate	10 each leg	Consecutive
Crisscross	90	Intermediate	5 each leg	Alternating
Leg Pull	138	Advanced	5	Use modification
Seal	102	Intermediate	5	

Table 10.3 Advanced Pilates Program

Exercise	Page number	Level	Repetitions	Comments
Pelvic Curl	52	Fundamental	5	
Chest Lift	54	Fundamental	10	
Spine Twist Supine	62	Fundamental	5 each side	Alternating
Chest Lift With Rotation	64	Fundamental	5 each side	Alternating
Leg Lift Side	58	Fundamental	10	Both exercises on same side; switch sides and repeat
Leg Pull Side	60	Fundamental	10	
Back Extension Prone	66	Fundamental	5	
One-Leg Circle	70	Fundamental	5 each leg	Alternating
Hundred	78	Intermediate	10 breath cycles	
Roll-Up	73	Intermediate	5	
Rolling Back	100	Fundamental	10	
Spine Stretch	98	Fundamental	5	
Rocker With Open Legs	108	Intermediate	5	
Shoulder Bridge	128	Intermediate	5 each leg	Consecutive
Single Straight-Leg Stretch	84	Intermediate	5 each leg	Alternating
Double-Leg Stretch	87	Intermediate	10	
Saw	161	Intermediate	5 each side	Alternating
Spine Twist	158	Intermediate	5 each side	Alternating
Rollover With Legs Spread	112	Advanced	6	
Control Balance	120	Advanced	3 each leg	Alternating
One-Leg Kick	178	Intermediate	10 each leg	Alternating
Double Kick	181	Intermediate	6	
Cat Stretch	176	Fundamental	5	
Scissors	131	Advanced	5 each leg	Alternating
Bicycle	134	Advanced	5 each leg	Alternating
Crisscross	90	Intermediate	5 each leg	Alternating
Corkscrew	168	Advanced	3 each side	Alternating
Jackknife	123	Advanced	5	
Hip Twist With Stretched Arms	171	Advanced	3 each side	Alternating
Leg Pull Front	142	Intermediate	5 each leg	Alternating
Push-Up	145	Advanced	5	

Exercise	Page number	Level	Repetitions	Comments
Swimming	184	Intermediate	10 breath cycles	
Side Kick Kneeling	152	Intermediate	10 each leg	Both exercises on same side; switch sides and repeat
Side Bend	154	Advanced	5 each side	
Teaser	92	Advanced	5	
Leg Pull	138	Advanced	5 each leg	Alternating
Boomerang	116	Advanced	3 each leg	Alternating
Crab	104	Advanced	6	
Rocking	187	Advanced	5	
Seal	102	Intermediate	5	

which often use the hip, back, and shoulder extensors, provide necessary balance. Foundation (warm-up) and abdominal work use primarily the flexors, so bridging exercises are a welcome change in both muscle focus and direction of motion. Alternating from flexion to extension and vice versa is a consistent element in the work of Joseph Pilates. Exercises for the sides of the body are important for all activities, whether everyday, recreational, or professional. Finally, back extension should be included in every program, if at all possible. The importance of this category cannot be overemphasized and has been discussed in greater depth in chapter 9. Modern society, with all its wonders, has led to certain postural and alignment ills, such as round shoulders and weak upper backs. A strong back can help remedy these imbalances and prevent the repercussions that arise from them.

The sample programs provided are of varying levels and draw appropriate exercises from each chapter. When beginning a program, start with exercises noted as fundamental that are suitable for your current fitness and health. Omit any exercises that cause discomfort or that are contraindicated for you. Prepare your body well for each new exercise and for the more advanced programs. As your skill increases, gradually add intermediate-level and then advanced-level exercises. This will allow improvement, challenge, and variety. As you progress and your control improves, increase ranges of motion and try variations. In Pilates, making an exercise more difficult often does not equate to greater strength demands (increased resistance) but instead relates more closely to neuromuscular coordination and timing. Remember, this process takes time and much practice. Work up to these programs and then beyond. Do not rush, for the process itself is so valuable and beneficial. View this as a lifelong journey and part of your commitment to well-being.

Many of the more challenging exercises include modifications, and you may need to use them. Do not limit yourself to just these modifications. If needed, seek professional advice to help create ones that are optimal for your body. Creating modifications demands knowledge of the human body, knowledge of the exercises, awareness of restrictions and medical history, and a great deal of creativity. It is a very exciting aspect of Pilates practice. For this reason, it is highly recommended that you work with a teacher and continue with regular self-practice, no matter what your level.

Finally, remember that the programs offered are only samples. They should be practiced, mastered, enjoyed, and ultimately changed around, keeping your practice fresh, challenging, and fun.

BIBLIOGRAPHY

Suggested Readings

Clippinger, K. 2007. *Dance anatomy and kinesiology.* Champaign, IL: Human Kinetics.

Isacowitz, R. 2006. *Pilates.* Champaign, IL: Human Kinetics.

Pilates, J., and Miller, W. 2003. *Return to life through contrology.* Miami: Pilates Method Alliance.

Additional References and Resources

American College of Sports Medicine. 2010. *ACSM's resource manual for guidelines for exercise testing and prescription.* Philadelphia: Lippincott Williams & Wilkins.

Axler, C., and McGill, S. 1997. Low back loads over a variety of abdominal exercises: Searching for the safest abdominal challenge. *Medicine & Science in Sports & Exercise* 29(6):804-810.

Balanced Body Pilates. Pilates origins. Available: www.pilates.com/BBAPP/V/pilates/origins-of-pilates.html.

Briggs, A., van Dieën, J., Wrigley, T., Greig, A., Phillips, B., Lo, S., and Bennell, K. 2007. Thoracic kyphosis affects spinal loads and trunk muscle force. *Physical Therapy* 87(5):595-607.

Carpenter, D., Graves, J., Pollock, M., Leggett, S., Foster, D., Holmes, B., and Fulton, M. 1990. Effect of 12 and 20 weeks of training on lumbar extension strength (abstract). *Medicine & Science in Sports & Exercise* (supplement) 22(2):S19.

Clippinger, K. 2002. Complementary use of open and closed kinetic chain exercises. *Journal of Dance Medicine and Science* 6(3):77-78.

Cools, M., Witvrouw, E., Declercq, G., Danneels, L., and Cambier, D. 2003. Scapular muscle recruitment patterns: Trapezius muscle latency with and without impingement symptoms. *American Journal of Sports Medicine* 31:542-549.

Csíkszentmihályi, M. 1990. *Flow: The psychology of optimal experience.* New York: Harper & Row.

De Troyer, A., Estenne, M., Ninane, V., Gansbeke, D., and Gorini, M. 1990. Transversus abdominis muscle function in humans. *Journal of Applied Physiology* 68(3):1010-1016.

Fletcher, Ron. 2010. Personal communication regarding percussive breathing. February 14, 2010.

Friedman, P., and Eisen, G. 1980. *The Pilates method of physical and mental conditioning.* New York: Warner Books.

Gallagher, S., and Kryzanowskka, R. 1999. *Pilates method of body conditioning.* Philadelphia: Bainbridge Books.

Hamill, J., and Knutzen, K. 2009. *Biomechanical basis of human movement.* Philadelphia: Lippincott Williams & Wilkins.

Kendall, F., McCreary, E., and Provance, P. 1993. *Muscles: Testing and function.* Baltimore: Williams & Wilkins.

Kincade, J., Dougherty, M., Carlson, J., and Wells, E. 2007. Factors related to urinary incontinence in community-dwelling women. *Urologic Nursing* 27(4):307-317.

Kincade, J., Dougherty, M., Busby-Whitehead, J., Carlson, J., Nix, W., Kelsey, D., Smith, F., Hunter, G., and Rix, A. 2005. Self-monitoring and pelvic floor muscle exercises to treat urinary incontinence. *Urologic Nursing* 25(5):353-363.

Kreighbaum, E., and Barthels, K. 1996. *Biomechanics: A qualitative approach for studying human movement.* Boston: Allyn and Bacon.

Levangie, P., and Norkin, C. 2001. *Joint structure and function: A comprehensive analysis.* Philadelphia: Davis.

Marieb, E., and Hoehn, K. 2006. *Human anatomy and physiology.* New York: Pearson /Benjamin Cummings.

Moore, K., and Dalley, A. 1999. *Clinically oriented anatomy.* Philadelphia: Lippincott Williams & Wilkins.

Moseley, M., Jobe, F., Pink, M., Perry, J., and Tibone, J. 1992. EMG analysis of the scapular muscles during a shoulder rehabilitation program. *American Journal of Sports Medicine* 20(2):128-134.

Otis, C. 2009. *Kinesiology: The mechanics and pathomechanics of human movement.* Philadelphia: Lippincott Williams & Wilkins.

Richardson, C., Hodges, P., and Hides, J. 2004. *Therapeutic exercise for lumbopelvic stabilization.* London: Churchill Livingstone.

Sapsford, R., and Hodges, P. 2001. Contraction of the pelvic floor muscles during abdominal maneuvers. *Archives of Physical Medicine and Rehabilitation* 82:1081-1088.

Siler, B. 2000. *The Pilates body.* New York: Broadway Books.

Wilmore, J., and Costill, D. 2004. *Physiology of sport and exercise.* Champaign, IL: Human Kinetics.

EXERCISE FINDER

Side Exercises for an Effective Core

Extensions for a Strong Back

*Exercises not appearing in Joseph Pilates' *Return to Life Through Contrology*.

ABOUT THE AUTHORS

Rael Isacowitz is a world-renowned practitioner and teacher of Pilates. He has over 30 years of Pilates achievement and is a prominent lecturer and teacher at symposiums, universities, and studios around the globe.

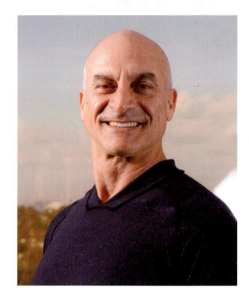

Rael earned his bachelor of education degree from the Wingate Institute, Israel, and holds a master of arts degree in dance from the University of Surrey, England. During his career he has worked with numerous Olympians and many professional athletes and dancers.

Rael's early Pilates teachers included Alan Herdman and thereafter several of the first-generation Pilates teachers (known as the Elders). To Kathy Grant, Ron Fletcher, Romana Kryzanowska, Eve Gentry, and Lolita San Miguel, Rael owes the inspiration and friendship that have guided his career.

Rael has mastered all levels of the Pilates repertoire and is noted for his unique athleticism and passion for teaching as well as his synthesis of body, mind, and spirit. In 1989, he founded Body Arts and Science International (BASI Pilates), which has developed into one of the foremost Pilates education organizations in the world. At present, BASI Pilates is represented in 20 countries.

Rael has authored the definitive book on Pilates (*Pilates,* Human Kinetics), published a series of training manuals on all the Pilates apparatus, produced DVDs, designed the revolutionary Avalon equipment, and created *Pilates Interactive,* the groundbreaking Pilates software. He is a regular contributor to several industry publications. Creativity and energy suffuse his work. For Rael, teaching Pilates is the ultimate gift. Isacowitz resides in Hood River, Oregon.

Karen Clippinger is a professor at California State University at Long Beach, where she teaches functional anatomy for dance, body placement, Pilates, and other dance science courses. She is also on the faculty for Body Arts and Science International (BASI Pilates), where she teaches Pilates certification programs. Furthermore, she teaches continuing education courses for BASI Pilates and other prominent organizations.

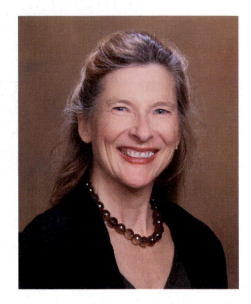

Ms. Clippinger holds a master's degree in exercise science. Her lifelong passion is to make anatomical and biomechanical principles accessible so that people can better understand their bodies, improve technique, and prevent injuries. Her textbook, *Dance Anatomy and Kinesiology*, exemplifies this mission; reviewers have lauded the book for its combination of scientific comprehensiveness and practical wisdom.

Before joining academia, Clippinger worked as a clinical kinesiologist for 22 years at Loma Linda University Medical Center and several sports medicine clinics in Seattle, Washington. She has worked with hundreds of professional dancers and elite athletes and consulted for the U.S. Weightlifting Federation, U.S. race walking team, Pacific Northwest Ballet, and California Governor's Council on Physical Fitness and Sports. During that time she was drawn to Pilates because of its tremendous versatility and profound benefits for people of varying abilities and aspirations.

Clippinger is a renowned presenter in Pilates, dance, anatomy, and biomechanics. She has given more than 375 presentations throughout the United States and in Australia, Canada, England, Japan, New Zealand, and South Africa. Clippinger was also an exercise columnist for *Shape* magazine for four years. She resides in Long Beach, California.

ANATOMY SERIES

Each book in the *Anatomy Series* provides detailed, full-color anatomical illustrations of the muscles in action and step-by-step instructions that detail perfect technique and form for each pose, exercise, movement, stretch, and stroke.

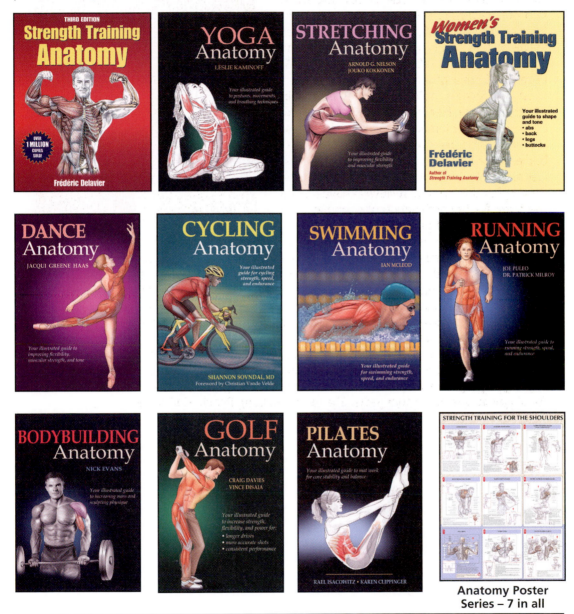

Anatomy Poster Series – 7 in all

HUMAN KINETICS
The Premier Publisher for Sports & Fitness
P.O. Box 5076, Champaign, IL 61825-5076